Why *Not* Me?
Oh God
Why *Me*?

Why *Not* Me?
Oh God
Why *Me?*

✦

One Woman's Inspirational and Thought-provoking Journey with God through Cancer

Sue Teall

iUniverse, Inc.
New York Lincoln Shanghai

Why *Not* Me? Oh God Why *Me?*
One Woman's Inspirational and Thought-provoking Journey with God through Cancer

Copyright © 2007 by Sue Teall

iUniverse books may be ordered through booksellers or by contacting:

iUniverse
2021 Pine Lake Road, Suite 100
Lincoln, NE 68512
www.iuniverse.com
1-800-Authors (1-800-288-4677)

Because of the dynamic nature of the Internet, any Web addresses or links contained in this book may have changed since publication and may no longer be valid.

The views expressed in this work are solely those of the author and do not necessarily reflect the views of the publisher, and the publisher hereby disclaims any responsibility for them.

Scripture verses are from the NIV Life Application Bible—Zondervan

ISBN: 978-0-595-43675-0 (pbk)
ISBN: 978-0-595-88004-1 (ebk)

Printed in the United States of America

Lovingly dedicated to my three grandsons

Jacob, Joshua, and Justin

Who enhance my life with laughter

And beautiful rays of sunshine

Contents

Foreword

Comfort is most comfortable when its source is experience.

Sue Teall has allowed herself the activation of memory in order to offer comfort. The exercise of Faith and the deliberation of Hope punctuate the story of her journey and will leave stepping-stones to the path others will follow.

Jeannette Clift George

Founder and Artistic Director of the
A.D. Players and Published Writer

Preface

I am speaking to my niece, Linda Ravencraft, on the phone. She is enjoying a beautiful, new faith journey with God and loves to share her excitement and joy with me. It is May 2001, and I have been a statistic with breast cancer for about three months. She is one of many people who receive frequent e-mails from me regarding my journey with cancer and with God.

Linda: "Aunt Susan, you do understand God's purpose for you while you plod along on this incredible trek, don't you?"

Me: "I'm not sure, Lin. Why don't you tell me?"

Linda: "Well, duh! You would never reveal so openly and intimately and profoundly your relationship with God if it weren't for the cancer updates you send to so many people via the e-mail. Don't you see that the cancer is the vehicle which God is using for you to reveal him and how he has been a blessing in your life? God offers love and hope to all of us who read your e-mails. It's your mission, Aunt Susan. Don't you see that?"

Me: "Is that how you truly see it?"

Linda: "Yeah! That's how I see it."

We end our conversation and I smile at her insight. She just expressed what I have clearly sensed God saying to me from the inception of this journey. How awesome that God might use my cancer experience to reveal himself to others! God does work in mysterious ways. With deepest humility, I hope and pray that his love and his power and his grace will be reflected in my story.

1

It Could Happen to Me

I have always been responsible (my husband Dave would say paranoid) about my own health concerns. I admit to a certain anxiety and perhaps some tension and just a bit of fear over the years as I experienced a variety of health issues and nuisances. After all, I was raised by parents who overreacted rather quickly to any symptoms of illness displayed by my sister Karen, my brother Jeff, or me, by calling the family doctor for advice or—preferably—a quick house call in the evening when I am sure he would have rather been home stroking his dog.

So it follows that I am very religious in having yearly checkups by my gynecologist and primary care physician. I have been faithful with pap smears, mammograms, blood tests, dermatology exams, and the like. But in my so-called paranoia, I was more concerned with heart-related issues, osteoporosis, and Alzheimer's, to which I have a genetic predisposition. My mother suffered from serious dementia and died of a massive heart attack. My father had three heart attacks and triple bypass surgery. Karen and Jeff have both been on blood pressure and cholesterol medications for many years. Cancer seemed very remote. Therefore, I was not very consistent at doing self breast exams. But what did it matter? After all, my gynecologist was checking me in the summer and my primary care physician was checking me in the winter. Surely, with all of this medical attention, I had no need to be concerned.

The phone rang one steamy August morning in the year 2000. I was thrilled to hear the voice of my dear friend, Ronnie. She and her husband, Bob, live in Florida, so we don't get to see each other as often as we did when she lived in Houston. Ronnie and I have shared much laughter over the years. We joke about our chubby cheeks and how they keep the wrinkles away. We rarely try to solve the world's problems, but we sure do elevate each other's sense of fun. I am always happy to be sharing a conversation with Ronnie.

****

I asked God to lead my prayer, and he did.

****

But this day was different. Ronnie wasn't her jovial self. She immediately asked me if I would pray for her as she had just been diagnosed with breast cancer. My body tensed; I was shocked, saddened, and frightened for her. I'm sure I said some rather meaningless words as she explained her situation. Suddenly, I felt a need to pray for her right then and I asked if that was okay. Silently, I asked God to lead my prayer, and he did. I thanked him for his grace and mercy, and for Ronnie. I asked for his comfort, his peace, his healing, and his love for Ronnie and for Bob. Ronnie thanked me, and I felt we both knew that God's presence was with us. The last thing she said to me was, "Do your breast self-exams."

When we hung up, tears fell down my cheeks. I just wanted Ronnie to be okay. My heart went out to her as I imagined the trauma she would be experiencing over the next many months. I felt alone and confused and, suddenly, scared. If it could happen to Ronnie, it could happen to me. I vowed to myself that I was going to do monthly self-exams from that day forward. And I did. Six months to the day of Ronnie's phone call, I was in the shower and I felt the lump.

2

No Big Deal—Or Is It?

Showers for me are generally times of relaxation, meditation, prayer, or just concentrated thought. Perhaps that morning I was thinking about my older son Mike and his wife, Marla, who were about to celebrate their fourth wedding anniversary, and how delighted Dave and I were to be a part of their lives and watch them parent their twenty-one-month-old son, Jake, with such love and joy and wonderment. Or maybe I was deciding what to pack for a weeklong trip to Scottsdale, Arizona, which Dave and I were anticipating in just a few days. Or perhaps I was simply giving thanks to God for the prospect of a new day.

****

Suddenly I froze! "What the heck is that?"
****

I don't remember if I was doing an intentional breast check, or just soaping my body. Suddenly, I froze! "What the heck is that?" I skimmed my fingers over my left breast several times. I couldn't believe it! There was a solid lump beneath my fingertips, just to the left of the nipple. I stopped touching it and just stood there in disbelief, letting the warm water slither down my body. My mind was racing in a thousand different directions. Anything that I might have been focused on just a moment before was lost; my total attention was centered on this foreign object that had not been there the last time I checked. "Maybe it will just disappear if I don't touch it?" But I did touch it again. And it hadn't disappeared.

"How can this be?" Panic began to envelop me. Then I remembered that twenty-three years before, I had a similar experience in which the lump thankfully was determined to be a benign cyst. The tension and the fear began to subside as I recalled that my mother had experienced several benign cysts over the years. Even I had endured three or four simple surgical procedures in the past to remove benign cysts from my back and arm. "No big deal," I concluded. I

3

decided I would simply wait for three days to see my primary care physician, Dr. Roger Schultz, at an appointment already scheduled for a routine yearly exam.

Upon completion of the general exam, Dr. Schultz asked if I wanted a breast check. I affirmed that I did, but I hadn't told him about my discovery. I was carefully watching his expression as he proceeded to examine my left breast. He indicated that he felt a lump, which I then revealed I knew was there. He suggested I have a mammogram, but he wasn't convinced it was anything to worry about. I told him I would get the mammogram through my gynecologist as all my previous records were with him.

That very day I called for an appointment, and was told it would be eight days before I could be scheduled. Dave and I decided that as long as I couldn't be scheduled immediately, we would go on our trip to Scottsdale, and upon the approval of my gynecologist, I made the appointment for eleven days hence. Three extra days would be of no significance. And besides, I really wasn't all that concerned.

Scottsdale was lovely. In the mornings, the desert golf course was awash with dew and even frost. By 9:00 AM the sun was in control, the skies were a perfect blue, the fairways were lush, and the desert air was so refreshing. We enjoyed three mornings of solitude as we played golf surrounded by the beauty of the desert hills. I felt serene and blessed and very grateful for this time away from thoughts of the lump. We dodged snow flakes on a side trip to Sedona, we laughed a lot, we enjoyed the art galleries and wonderful restaurants, and we celebrated Dave's fifty-eighth birthday on Valentine's Day. Any notion of the potential seriousness of my situation just didn't surface to a conscious level for either of us.

The results of the mammogram were suspect. My gynecologist, Dr. Gary Urano, ordered an ultrasound for the following morning. I was beginning to sense uneasiness, and shared my concern that evening at a weekly Bible study with seven other women from my church. This group had been the brainchild of a dear friend of mine, Susan, and her very close friend, Mary Kent. Two months before, Susan and I had shared lunch at her beautifully decorated home during the Christmas season. She explained that she and Mary Kent desired to bring eight women of faith together each week for meaningful worship, study, prayer, and fellowship. She shared the names of the other women and then invited me to be one of them.

I took a moment to silently pray about the opportunity and the commitment. I felt somewhat intimidated by these women whom I knew by reputation to be very strong and articulate in their faith. But I had been missing this component in my life for some time, and as I sensed God urging me to accept this invitation,

I had no idea that he would use this group to be such a spiritual and loving support over the next year. I simply accepted the invitation and thanked God for this amazing opportunity. We met for the first time in late January—just ten days before I found the lump.

Dave went with me for the ultrasound. As I was being examined, I kept my eyes closed and tried to focus on God. I prayed silently, recognizing God's sovereignty, yet asking that this test would eliminate any further concern. That was not to be. I was told to call Dr. Urano and have him order a biopsy, which he did for that same morning. My fears were beginning to entrap me. I remember clearly thinking, in the sterile environment of that testing room, that I just wanted to leave and forget that this potential nightmare was even happening. Instead, I was prepped for the needle biopsy. I was told it would be a couple of days before the results were known.

It was a very quiet drive home. Neither Dave nor I knew what to say. Dave, in his optimistic manner, tried to be encouraging, but by now, in the very deepest part of my being, I feared the results would prove malignancy.

3

Why Not Me?

Please God, no! Please, please, no! My desperate plea seemed to be echoing against deaf ears. I was so afraid! I was pacing, alone in my home waiting for the phone to ring. My knees were weak and my heart was racing. Fear gripped my every thought and every part of my being. Oh, God, please, no!

As I looked out my window on that beautiful February morning filled with sunshine and cool crisp air, I watched the birds eating at our bird feeder outside the window. It all seemed so surreal. The turmoil I was going through was so agitated against the backdrop of that serene picture of a male and female cardinal, in their glorious splendor, seemingly enjoying the beauty of the day.

Dave had been delayed at the dentist's office. I was alone—alone with my anxiety, my desperate plea, yet sensing deep in my soul that I already knew the answer. When the phone rang, I nervously picked up the receiver and listened as the nurse on the other end told me she hated to be the bearer of bad news, but the results of the biopsy determined that I did indeed have breast cancer. I sensed her warmth and compassion, and I thanked her for telling me in such a kind way.

****

I said aloud, "Why *not* me?"
****

While this conversation was unfolding, something incredible and miraculous was also happening to me. As she told me the dreaded news, the most amazing peace and calm washed over my entire body. I was no longer frightened! I was no longer weak with fear and anxiety! Instead, I felt the loving arms of God enfold me and comfort me and assure me that I was not alone. I knew that God was telling me that he would be with me every step of the journey that lay ahead. I sat down, bowed my head and thanked God for his love and mercy and compassion. I wasn't sure what was in store for me, but I just knew deep in my soul, where

God's voice is often so clear, that we would get through this ordeal and come out whole on the other end. I just wasn't sure what the other end would look like.

I said aloud, "Why *not* me?" Women hear this news every day of the week. Why would I ever think that I was so special that I too would not suffer the ordeal of cancer?

Dave walked through the door. As our eyes met, the tears calmly rolled down my cheeks. He knew. We didn't speak. He simply came to me and wrapped his arms around me. We stood there for several moments as our tears joined together and we let the reality sink in. For the incredible truth was that I had cancer, and our lives were about to change for a very long time.

4

God Had Prepared Me

The Bible tells us in Philippians 4:7, "And the peace of God, which transcends all understanding, will guard your hearts and your minds in Christ Jesus." At the very moment that I was being told my body had been invaded by cancer, the incredible peace of God enveloped my heart, my soul, and my mind, bathing me in soothing tranquility. The predicted behavior (from past history dealing with my own health issues) would have found me hysterical, frightened, panicked, and totally out of control. But the God who loves me beyond comprehension, the God who has forgiven my every transgression, the God who yearns to have me walk alongside him—this God, whom I love and worship and trust, intervened and offered me his gracious peace.

I do not believe for one moment that God caused me to have cancer. I know that he allows pain and suffering and tragedy on this earth, and I believe that in his sovereignty and omniscience God knows exactly what will happen to each of us as we meander through a lifetime in a world that is filled with imperfection. I believe he weeps with us when we weep and laughs with us in our joy! And I believe that he had been preparing me for this moment over the span of my life.

****

... the incredible peace of God enveloped my heart, my soul, and my mind ...
****

I was baptized into the Presbyterian Church when I was an infant. It was my mother's simple faith and strong will that Karen, Jeff, and I would be raised in Sunday school and church. Although I never saw my mother read the Bible, and I rarely heard her pray, deep in my heart I knew that she loved God. My father attended church on Christmas and Easter and graciously referred to God as "the man upstairs." Because we rarely talked about prayer or faith or spirituality or even God, there was little depth to my Christian upbringing. Still, somehow I knew that I was very connected to God.

Dave had also grown up in the Presbyterian Church. When we married in 1965 and eventually had two beautiful sons, there was never a doubt that we would raise Mike and Jim in the same manner and tradition to which we were accustomed. We went to Sunday school and church as part of our weekly routine. The boys attended vacation Bible studies and church activities. Dave and I both were very active in the life of the church and had numerous roles of leadership through the years.

In 1993, our younger son Jim was earnestly seeking God's will as to whether he was being called into ministry. He and I had many wonderful conversations about God and religion and theology. During the course of one of these conversations, Jim courageously and lovingly told me that he didn't think I understood the real meaning of being a Christian. I sat there in total shock! I was dumbfounded that this twenty-five-year-old son of mine could even fathom that I was naïve about Christianity. I vehemently defended myself. "Jim," I said, "how can you possibly say that? I've been involved with the Presbyterian Church my entire life. I've taught Sunday school, faithfully attended worship, and have served on many committees. I've volunteered in community projects for years and even led your first missionary trip to Mexico. I am an elder;[1] I've served on two church staffs and had many accomplishments in those positions. What are you talking about?" Jim listened quietly, and then said, "Mom, you have not said one word about prayer, or faith, or the Bible, or even Christ. Your Christianity is based upon what you have accomplished."

This time the shock was the incredible revelation of truth which Jim had just exposed to me! Using our son as the vehicle, God was about to radically turn my so-called Christian life upside down. I began to reflect on my past and recognized the shallowness of my spiritual life—our spiritual life as a family. Yes, we went to church, but we never discussed the scripture reading or the sermon. We didn't read the Bible, although each of us had one that sat on the shelf and collected dust. Occasionally we said grace before a special dinner, but our prayers as a family had been when the children were little and we repeated the "Now I lay me down to sleep" prayer. My own prayers were generally said when I was desperate for God to fulfill a need for me or my family.

Sure, I had accomplished a great deal over the years in the name of God and the church, but I had been missing the essence of what it means to be in relationship with God through Jesus Christ. My life and our family life had not been focused on God. It became clear that our family behaviors were independently

---

1.   A member of the ruling body of the Presbyterian Church

selfish, worldly, and not in sync with God's will. I was deeply saddened and full of shame and regret for opportunities missed in the guidance of my children toward the Lord. Yet here was the God of forgiveness offering me a new journey—one that would temporarily remove me from the role of Martha, the doer, and guide me into the role of Mary, the seeker of God's revealing word (Luke 10:38-42).

****

I basked in my newly found relationship with Christ.

****

I was ecstatic as I began my journey to see God more clearly, to follow his guidance, and to love and trust him through his word in the Bible. I learned the discipline of unselfish prayers of praise, confession, thanksgiving, and intercession. I attended Bible studies, read incessantly the works of Christian writers and theologians, listened to praise and worship music and the wonderful old hymns. I basked in my newly found relationship with Christ. I had no idea during those times how much I was going to draw on the strength and truth of God's faithfulness, and of my ever growing faith just a few years hence, when I would be diagnosed with cancer.

5

Praise God for My Family

Mike, Marla, and Jim had been aware that I had a lump and was going through the tests. Yet it was a difficult moment for me and for them when I spoke the words, "The results came back, and I do have cancer." Although I was calm and hopeful, it was a moment of realization for all of us that I could die. What is it about the reality of death that elicits such fright in the depths of our being? After all, death for a Christian is the ultimate moment of glory when we come face-to-face with God! What could be more wonderful and joyous than that? However, at the very moment of verbalizing the dreaded truth to my children, there was a deep sadness and fear among all of us. I was so touched by their supportive words. I wrote that night in my journal, "I feel so blessed to have my family. I am overcome with Dave's love and tenderness and the genuine feelings of love and support from Mike and Marla and Jim."

We discussed whether and how to communicate the information to friends and family. I have found that each person who is diagnosed with this ugly disease responds to the dilemma in very different ways. Many want the privacy of as few people as possible knowing what they are enduring. It is such a personal and intimate decision. As I debated the issue, I asked God for direction. It was so clear to me that God was going to use my cancer journey in ways that would reflect his power and his compassion and his great love. And I was convinced that as he journeyed with me over the next many months, I was to share him through my story. That night Jim and Dave each wrote an e-mail to some two hundred people around the world alerting them to my situation and seeking their prayers.

6

Everything Has Changed—Nothing Has Changed

It is Thursday, February 22. I have known for a full twenty-four hours that I have a cancer that is growing at will in my body. I prepare breakfast and make the bed and do a load of laundry and go to the grocery store as if nothing is wrong. It feels like an out-of-body experience. I know it is true; everything has changed and nothing has changed. It's almost as if it is happening to someone else. How strange!

Dave made arrangements through Shell Oil Company, with which he was employed for thirty-two years and from which he is now retired. Shell has an insurance agreement with MD Anderson Cancer Institute located in Houston. Today I am enrolled as a patient in a place which will soon become very familiar and encouraging for me. MD Anderson has been consistently ranked as the leader of all cancer facilities in the United States. How fortunate to be in Houston at this moment of my life! Dave and I reflect on the events that brought us here and smile at the mysterious ways God guides and directs our lives even when we are unaware.

Dave's entire career had been in Human Resources at Shell locations in many parts of the country including Houston from 1977 to 1988. In 1997, we had been living in New Orleans for nine years. We were fifty-four years old, and at that time he was planning to work about five or six more years. Then we would consider retiring in North Carolina. One day he came home from the office and indicated that there was a job in Houston which intrigued him from a professional standpoint, but not location-wise. Dave didn't particularly want to go back to Houston. A few days later, he told me that he couldn't seem to dismiss from his mind this job that had not yet been filled, and that he felt compelled to place his name in contention even though it was not in his career field and he had been advised that if he left Human Resources for a few years, there probably would not be a job available back in his field at a later time. He posted for the job. Shortly thereafter, he called from the office and said, "Pack your bags; we're moving to Houston." I was very excited as we had a newly-married son, some extended family, and many friends in a city which I had previously enjoyed as home.

Dave's new job was as a member of the corporate Business Transformation Team (BTT), which was formed by the CEO to help change the culture and focus of the company. The members of the team were representative of various components of the business and were brought together to learn new ways in which to manage a major corporation as a team, and then help implement these ideas through the senior staff. The irony of the situation was that it was the "curriculum of the job itself" which precipitated Dave's retirement and complete change of heart and purpose for his life.

During one segment of a six-week seminar which was held in the mountains of Colorado, the focus was getting in touch with yourself and pondering your priorities. Dave went off by himself, and while sitting on the crest of a mountain viewing the splendor of God's creation, reflecting on his past and pondering his future, he felt God hold him in the palm of his hand and literally move his body forward. He was stunned! He was incredulous! He wept! He understood that God was urging him in a new direction that would put serving God and his family at the focus of his life rather than the pursuit of money and career. He retired within months at the age of fifty-five.

****

... God guides and directs our lives even when we are unaware.

****

So here we are on this February day, delighted that we are in Houston. Soon I will be entrenched at MD Anderson. Dave is free from corporate responsibilities and can readily take charge of arrangements for me and be my faithful support system for the journey that lies ahead.

We made two very special visits that day which buoyed my hope and resolve. First, we saw our grandson Jake, at his day care. He brings me such wonderful joy. He jumped into my arms and we held each other so tightly. He seemed to cling to me as if he knew he was a special source of comfort and strength to me. And he is!

Then we went to church and visited with Asa Hunt, the associate pastor at First Presbyterian Church of Houston. Asa is a dear friend, and he shared the news that eighteen years ago, his wife experienced the same trauma. He told us that this cancer was not just mine, but Dave's also. We were to be in this absolutely together. He also told Dave that he couldn't fix the problem, so not to try. He said, "Just let her speak freely, cry freely, lament freely without words of admonishment, judgment or solution." How freeing for both of us! I told Asa that I didn't want to die—not so much because I feared death (although at that moment, I probably wasn't being totally truthful), but just because I wanted to live for my family and to serve God. He prayed with us and I felt the closeness of God through this humble, gentle servant.

Jim visited us later in the day and told us of the many responses to his e-mail from people who are lifting me to God in prayer. Dave and I could hardly speak. With tears in our eyes at the realization of the power those prayers invoked, we were overcome with humility and gratitude for this intervention by so many on my behalf. I hugged Jim and thanked him again for having the courage and the will to obey God a few years earlier when challenging my faith, and then to guide me to a deep and precious relationship with God on which I now could rely so intently. I wrote in my journal, "God is good!"

7

Oh, How Difficult Is the Waiting!

Waiting! Waiting! Waiting! Oh, how difficult is the waiting! As a society, we tend to abhor waiting for just about anything. Our fingers do a tap dance on the grocery cart when we pick the wrong line which seems to be moving in slow motion. We sigh impatiently when the computer seems to languish before giving us the information we seek. Road rage occurs far too often when lines of traffic are at a standstill or when the red light seems to take an eternity to change to green. We become impatient as persons on the other end of the phone put us on hold to answer other calls. How dare they! Our stress levels boil over as we wait, wait, wait!

While we were living in New Orleans, I was blessed to have as my Bible teacher, mentor, and dear friend, a woman of great faith and exceptional teaching ability who possessed a keen sense of reality in dealing with situations involving the stress of everyday waiting. Gwen would suggest that when we are stopped at a traffic light, we should look around and begin to pray for the first person we see. When stalled in the grocery line, we should lift to God the problems and concerns of the cashier and seek his blessings for that person. When our nerves are frayed from the interminable wait at the doctor's office, we should listen to a tape of praise and worship songs. I am always amazed at the calming effect these actions evoke when I follow Gwen's advice.

As the days of waiting for information from MD Anderson regarding an appointment and a doctor continued, I was able to manage my time and thoughts fairly well during the daylight hours. I worked on our income taxes, I had my hair cut, I was deeply touched and humbled by the e-mails, notes, cards, and phone calls from so many people offering advice, encouragement, comfort, love, and prayer support. I spoke often with family and friends. I cherished special moments with my family and found such peace in the laughter and innocence of Jake. Mike shared with misty eyes that he was especially sad when he thought of the bond between Jake and me. I hugged him, knowing what he really meant was, "I do not want you to die."

Dave and I listened to motivational tapes and I was encouraged to be a winner—not a victim. I eagerly went to my evening Bible class to be embraced by the tender care and deep intercessory prayer on my behalf from these women to whom I had been sent by God.

One evening I attended a lecture at my church by Jeannette Clift George, who is a gifted author, teacher, speaker, actress, and humble servant of God. Many years ago she portrayed the lead character in the movie about Corrie Ten Boom entitled *The Hiding Place*. But on this night she made me belly laugh until the tears were rolling down my cheeks. The next moment I was genuinely weeping and felt a cleansing of my body and soul as she shared her personal relationship with Christ and his incredible love for all of us. I felt joyful and renewed. I was so grateful!

****

"Don't throw out your party dresses!"
****

Her warmth, her humor, and her faith encouraged me to approach her after the conclusion of her speech. I asked her if she had tapes available that I could listen to over the next weeks and months to help me laugh as I endured the unknown journey through cancer. Humor and laughter are so important in facing a long-term disease, and I felt her spontaneous and contagious laughter would be a blessed tonic for me. She looked at me with such compassion, and in her humble and gracious manner, she gathered six or seven women around us, took my hands, and prayed for God's healing and comforting presence to surround me. I was touched by the depth of her words on my behalf. We all said, "Amen," and then she said, "Don't throw out your party dresses!" It was such a special moment in time—one which gave me joyous hope and encouragement. God had placed me in her presence at just the perfect moment.

So I passed the days with relative calm. But then there were the nights. Darkness and aloneness led to unsolicited thoughts and fears and "what ifs" regarding the spread of this uninvited violator into other parts of my body. For weeks I had been enduring a very mild sore throat which I attributed to post-nasal drip. I had had a recurring gnawing sensation in my upper abdomen over the past few months which was often relieved by Tums. My left shin bone was very tender to the touch—but had been that way for years. What is it about the darkness that allows doubt and negative thoughts to overcome the hope and the trust in the light of the day? Had the cancer infiltrated my bones or my throat or my stomach? The biopsy report had indicated that the breast cancer had invaded the nodes under my left arm. I couldn't stop the thoughts from coming: "Oh, my God, were these devastating and deadly cells traveling at random through my body? Why doesn't the phone ring? How much longer can I survive the waiting?" I was becoming overwhelmed with my unanswered questions and uncontrolled imagination.

What I didn't know was that Kevin White, a physicians' assistant at MD Anderson and a very good friend of Jim's, was intervening on my behalf with Dr. Massimo Cristofanilli, the oncologist Kevin wanted as my doctor. On February 27, the much awaited phone call came. I was to see Dr. Cristofanilli on Tuesday, March 6. I found out later that my appointment date was being scheduled for March 23, but that Kevin had been instrumental in arranging the earlier time. I never see Kevin without thanking him profusely for his assistance. I will always be grateful for his intervention.

8

The Cancer Continues to Grow

One more week to wait before seeing the oncologist. One more week to muddle through with the intrusive cancer in physical control. The medical battle had not yet begun, but the spiritual battle including my own profound faith, love from family and friends, and the support of so many prayer warriors was well under way.

I continued to record my experiences during the interminable week of waiting.

Wednesday, February 28—Ash Wednesday—the cancer continues to grow

As Dave and I lie on the floor holding hands listening to a tape about dying, I realize that I have never come to grips about my own death. A sudden butterfly begins to well up inside my abdomen, and my hands feel clammy. I really don't want to think about my own death. Not now—not today. I remember when my father died in October 1991, (eighteen months after my mother's death) being acutely aware that my siblings and I were now the next generation to grow older and die. That had been a strange and troubling moment of rude awakening for me. But this morning as we listen to these beautiful words about dying, I do not sense my own death.

This evening we went to church to celebrate Ash Wednesday. The service was lovely and I felt such calm and peace. As Asa drew the sign of the cross with ashes on my forehead, he said, "You are dust and to dust you shall return!" Asa and I smiled brilliantly at one another knowing how glorious that moment will be one day to rest eternally in the holy arms of God. Still, I sensed for the second time today that I will not die from this cancer.

My prayer this day is that God will continue to fill me as a vessel of love and that I will reflect his greatness and his mercy as I go through this journey with him.

Thursday, March 1—the cancer continues to grow

I slept well last night. My sleep patterns have been less than satisfactory for the past few years, so I am always grateful when I sleep well. At Thursday morning Bible class, the teacher shared that we, as Christians, are commanded by God, because of his amazing love and sacrifice for us, his forgiveness of our sins, and his promise of salvation and eternal life, to go into the world and proclaim his truth and grace. "The world is a hurting place," she said, "and for most people this life on earth offers so little!" She spoke about her sorrow and painful sadness for the poor people of India with whom she had had the opportunity to share the power of hope and light of the Gospel.

I remember my own feelings of deep sadness and compassion for the hordes of people we encountered in China living in deplorable conditions of poverty and seeming hopelessness. Sometimes we get angry with God for allowing the many kinds of suffering which are rampant in the lives of people everywhere. Yet often it is in the deepest of life's suffering that we become closest to God. The apostle Paul says that he wants to share in Christ's suffering, thereby becoming more like him in his crucifixion and resurrection (Philippians 3:10). Wow!

"Lord, I do not know to what extent I will suffer, but I humbly ask that I will sense community with others who suffer and that I will have compassion and be able to offer your comfort and grace to them. I pray for people everywhere who live in poverty, in fear, in conflict. I pray for the sick, the disenfranchised, the lonely, the oppressed, and the depressed. I pray for the light of Christ to be brought to every weary soul. Amen."

The Bible group showered me with cards, gifts, well wishes, hugs, and prayers. I am so touched and so very blessed. Thank you, Father God.

Friday, March 2—the cancer continues to grow … or does it?

In the hymn "Jesus Loves Me," we are told that when we are weak, God is strong. I am so blessed to have been led by God to turn my cancer journey over to him. Already I am witnessing his hand and his strength as we travel along this dark path which continues to be infiltrated by his light.

On Monday evening at my women's group, when Susan and Mary Kent suggested a prayer session with Teddie Wright, a Christian counselor who has the spiritual gift of healing, I had much trepidation. My only experience of "faith healers" was as characters in movies, and my reaction was always negative. But I do know that God uses people to whom he gives special gifts. Having recently taught a class at church with Dave on spiritual gifts, I knew that biblically, the gift of healing was legitimate. Was God opening a door? Were Susan's and Mary Kent's experiences with Teddie, and my deep trust in them as exceptional women of faith, the vehicles which God was utilizing to grant me this opportunity?

I agreed to the session, and today I experienced the most incredible, powerful, humbling encounter with the Holy Spirit through the awesome prayers of Teddie, Susan, Mary Kent, and the other members of my precious Bible study group—Jan, Laura, Jo, Beverly, and Lillian—along with Dave, Jim, and Marla. I could feel God's power resonate throughout my body. He intervened and spoke to me through the words of this beloved group of friends and family. I am moved beyond descriptive words by the power of prayer and the love that emanated around that room—love of God and love for each other. The great commandment which Christ gives to us is to love God with all of our hearts, all of our souls and all of our might, and then to love one another. That commandment was fulfilled in that room on this day. The tears that fall down my cheeks are tears of joy. I believe I will be healed.

Saturday, March 3—God is in control

Why did I have such a tormented night? The fear, the uncertainty, the aloneness, the contemplation of death seemed to overpower me. *I do not want to die!* How can I in one moment sense so strongly God's will that I will live and then so quickly allow the opposite thought to consume me? I am weak, oh Lord; please be my strength! I trust that you are with me, and yet kernels of doubt seep into my very soul. Oh, Lord, I am like the father in the Gospel of Mark when he pleads with Christ saying, "I believe, help my unbelief!" (Mark 9:24) With tears I pray this prayer. Amen.

Sunday, March 4—This is the day the Lord has made; I will rejoice and be glad in it!

A beautiful morning filled with God's glory and hope, and yet I weep in Dave's arms. The contrast of this splendid Sabbath Day with the darkness in my physical body is difficult to reconcile. The church service brings me a sense of comfort, and I sing with gusto the Lord's Prayer. "Our Father, which art in heaven, hallowed be thy name. Thy kingdom come, thy will be done, on Earth as it is in Heaven. Give us this day our daily bread, and forgive us our debts as we forgive our debtors. And lead us not into temptation, but deliver us from evil, for thine is the kingdom and the power and the glory forever—Amen."

That's it! "But deliver us from evil!" In the Greek, the word "evil" means "the evil one." It is the plan of the evil spirit to keep us separated from God. My doubts and my fears and my lack of belief come when I allow evil to penetrate my faith in God. "Oh, Lord, I need you to help me fight the cancer, but I especially need your ultimate power and strength to fend off the intrusion of Satan into my life!"

9

The Butterflies Wax and Wane

The day finally arrived (five weeks after I had initially discovered the lump) when Dave and I began our trek to and around MD Anderson, which would soon become frequent and familiar and routine. We were greeted so warmly by our patient advocate and other personnel who were full of questions, information, forms to be completed and the like. In the main lobby, a pianist was playing beautiful and familiar music which seemed to ease my tension. There was an air of warmth and laughter and calm in the bustle of people surrounding us. Yet my temporary wish to be in denial of why I was here versus the reality of the situation wandered around in my head. What was I doing in this cancer institute? Well, of course: I was a patient.

We were escorted to the Nellie B. Connelly Breast Clinic, where we were again warmly greeted by a breast cancer survivor volunteer who generated a feeling of welcome and hope. Other patients waiting to see their doctor smiled, offering encouragement, praising the care, the treatment, and the operation of MD Anderson. I couldn't help but look at the faces of these women as I tried to sense their inner turmoil and concerns and fears. I stared at a young woman whose hair was like peach fuzz just beginning to reappear. How will I feel going through each of the stages of this journey?

****
What was I doing in this cancer institute? Well, of course: I was a patient.
****

My reverie was interrupted when I heard my name being called by a nurse. The butterflies kicked in as she led us to a patient examination room. She was so friendly and personable. I liked her immediately and noticed her engagement ring. We talked about her upcoming wedding as she performed her duties. The butterflies subsided.

When she left the room, Dave and I were alone. He was reading pages of data which had been given to us. I just watched him and thanked God that he was with me today and in life. He hadn't always been there for me and for our children when his career seemed so often to be his first priority. Many heartaches had occurred for us over the years, when our family's needs had lost out to a business meeting or work brought home in the evenings. Tears came to my eyes in the sterility of the examination room as I reflected on Dave's words from the previous night. He told me how much he had always loved me and promised that he would be with me throughout this journey, that he would take care of me and be my earthly support. How blessed I am that Dave's relatively recent acceptance of Christ as his Lord and Savior has transformed his priorities.

As I heard the door begin to open, the butterflies of anxiety forced their way back. Dr. Massimo Cristofanilli entered the room with dignity, extending a warm greeting, a handshake, and a beautiful smile. I instantly felt rapport with him and liked his gentle demeanor. He told us that from the preliminary data of the original tests ordered by my gynecologist, it appeared that I had a Stage II (perhaps Stage III) ductile carcinoma with invasion into more than one lymph node. He indicated that he would be more specific about my condition in a few days after I underwent several more tests. He told us that the protocol would likely include several months of chemotherapy followed by surgery and then radiation. "How strange," I said. "Why don't you perform the surgery first?" Dr. Cristofanilli explained that they would be monitoring the tumor's reaction to the chemo, but in the meantime, the chemo would also be attacking any cancer cells which might have escaped the nodes and be wandering around my system.

****
… and God is in control.
****

We asked a few additional questions which he graciously answered, but we never discussed "my chances" or "percentages" of survival. My primary care physician and friend, Dr. Schultz, had previously suggested to me that there are only two numbers that matter—0% and 100%. "You're either going to live, or you're going to die—the other percentages do not apply to your particular set of circumstances, so they are not relevant." I appreciated his simplistic approach, so I never sought that particular data from Dr. Cristofanilli. When it was time to leave, I held the doctor's hand and said, "You do what you have to do, I'll do what I have to do, and God is in control." He smiled and we left feeling hopeful.

That evening I spoke with my sister Karen, who is a nurse, and her husband Nate, who is an orthopedic surgeon. Nate had lost his first wife to breast cancer and is well aware of the different protocols. He applauded MD Anderson's approach. I was encouraged that, as a surgeon, he approved of the use of chemo as the initial phase of treatment.

10

Unfamiliar Surroundings

Over the next week, we spent countless hours at MD Anderson. It was like being at a theme park riding the merry-go-round and the roller coaster. The facility is very large, and we got our exercise going around and around, searching for the particular areas where I was expected for various tests, classes, demonstrations, and appointments. My emotions vacillated between the anxiousness of the climb up, up, up the track of the roller coaster to the fear of the sudden drop. Sometimes I was laughing; other times I cried. Sometimes I was verbose in greeting patients and staff; other times I was quiet and withdrawn. Sometimes I was ecstatic to be surrounded by such professionalism and expertise; other times I just wanted to disappear!

I had a mammogram, an ultrasound, biopsies of the nodes under my left arm and neck, a CAT scan, a chest x-ray, a bone scan, and blood tests. I had learned that breast cancer metastasizes to the liver, lungs, brain, and bones. We already were aware that the cancer had spread to the nodes under my arm. These additional tests would determine if there was any further invasion.

I cannot give enough praise and gratitude to the staff for their kindness, their concern, their gentleness, their humor, their professionalism, and, of course, their encouragement. In some ways, this was the most difficult week of the journey. It was a week of uncertainty: unfamiliar surroundings, a new vocabulary, anticipation before each test, anxiety while waiting for the results. It was exhausting, but although it was emotionally draining, it was a time for meeting new friends.

Dave and I were sitting in a waiting room and focused on a couple who looked as lost and confused and anxious as we felt. We introduced ourselves to Vernon and Lilly. She had breast cancer as well, and they would be traveling weekly to MD Anderson from Louisiana for her treatments. We offered the use of our home to them if needed at any time, and we all vowed to stay in touch and support each other. We still do.

Another day, while waiting in the women's dressing area for a bone scan, several of us shared our status on the cancer ladder. I was the only neophyte. One woman had had to cease her cancer treatments several months earlier in order to undergo heart surgery. But now, with a smile on her face and a gleam in her eye, she was back fighting the cancer. I was amazed at the power in each story of courage and fortitude amidst so many disappointing setbacks. There was incredible faith in God, immense hope for their treatments, and genuine support for each of us in that room. A feeling of kinship emanated from one to the other—a bond that can only be understood by those who have or have had breast cancer.

****
My heart broke for her!
****

A woman was sitting apart from the rest of us. She was obviously praying and tears quietly fell down her cheeks. Inspired by the gracious spirit I had just encountered with the other women, I went over to her and touched her arm. She looked at me with sad but serene eyes. Her name was Suad, and she was from Kuwait. She had found a lump while she was pregnant with her third child, but her doctor dismissed it as related to pregnancy. When she was finally diagnosed with breast cancer, it had already spread to other parts of her body. She was very ill. She had spent the past three years in the United States at two different facilities, fighting for her life while her children were in Kuwait being raised by her mother. My heart broke for her! The pain of her illness was one thing, but to be separated from her children was unbearable. Fortunately, her husband was able to be with her in their lonely struggle in a foreign land. I took her hand and promised I would pray for her and for her family. We spoke on the phone over the next few months, boosting each other's morale. One day I ran into her and she looked great. She was making much progress. We laughed and hugged and wished each other well. In our own personal prayer, we thanked God for each other.

Glorious relief came for me each day as the phone would ring and I would be told that test after test was negative. I was overjoyed knowing that the cancer hadn't spread, yet humbled realizing that some of my new acquaintances hadn't received the same good news along their journeys.

On Sunday, March 11, Mike and Marla and Jake came to our home for dinner. Jake was entertaining us as usual with his delightful "chatter" and innocent laughter and fun antics. I was so into enjoying this precious moment. Mike stood next to me, and as we relished Jake's every breath, Mike proudly said with such love and tenderness, "Isn't he something?" I responded, "Do you really know how much I love and cherish that little child of yours?" He smiled and nodded his head. I continued, "Well, you are my child and I love you even more!" It was a revelation of unconditional love for both Mike and me. Past hurts, angers, disagreements, and disappointments had no relevance in that moment when time stood still. With misty eyes, we silently hugged.

11

Second Chances

The doorbell rang on Monday morning, and a bubbly delivery woman handed me a gorgeous bouquet of flowers. She said that she hoped I was celebrating something very special! I thanked her and closed the door. When I opened the card, it simply said, "We love you," and was signed, "Your Tapestry Girls." With tears in my eyes, I smiled to myself that as the woman who delivered this special gift had said, I truly was celebrating something very beautiful!

Tapestry is the name of a group of young mothers who meet each week at our church for Bible study, fellowship, support, and intimate sharing. I had the privilege of being affiliated with this group as teacher, facilitator, mentor, and friend. I loved these young women, who were so genuine in their honesty, their unconditional love and support for each other, their deep willingness to share the intimacies of their hearts, their faith, their doubts, their struggles, their fears and frustrations and joys of motherhood, their disappointments and elations of marriage.

Wisdom and common sense might suggest that the role of the older woman is to share insight with women of the next generation. Tapestry afforded me the opportunity to reflect both on areas in which, as a wife and mother, I had done well, and on areas in which I had been far less than perfect. Our grown sons have shared with Dave and me some of the negative patterns and realities of our family life which have influenced some of their perceptions and behaviors in their adult lives.

****
… he was a "precious child of God."
****

In a sense, Tapestry was God's venue for me to share my past experiences with these precious women, to encourage them, and to help them avoid falling into similar patterns which have produced difficulties for our sons. Mike had queried me in his early thirties why I had never told him that he was a "precious child of

God." After I told that story at Tapestry, several of the moms informed me that they had gone home and tenderly shared with their children that they were beloved children of God! The moms were beaming with joy when they shared how excited their children were to hear that joyful news.

Sometimes it is the little things we do or don't do, say or don't say, which have the most lasting impact on our children. I thank God that the Tapestry women allowed me to be a part of them. In so many ways I learned more from them than they ever learned from me. And so I stared at the array of beautiful flowers, remembering their beautiful faces and appreciating their deep concern for my condition. I realized that I truly was celebrating something very special: love, children, family, community of faith ... and second chances.

12

God Is Awesome

I was in awe! I did not speak a word because I did not want the moment to be interrupted. I wished the phenomenon would remain, but I knew that would not be so. We were driving to MD Anderson for all-day appointments, and suddenly I gazed into the sky to witness this incredible sight the likes of which I had never seen before or since. In my heart I knew that it was a sign from God that he is ever-present with me and that I should not fear.

****
… the love of God had permeated my soul anew.
****

The dawn of that beautiful morning brought a perfectly gorgeous blue sky interspersed with billowy white clouds that looked like mounds of soft cotton. For the briefest of moments, one of the clouds began to open and slowly revealed the most amazing array of every color of the rainbow meandering through the fluffy white backdrop. The hues were vibrant and alive, and my heart felt full of joy. And then it was gone—swallowed up by the gentle movement of the journeying cloud formations across the sky. I silently said, "Yes! Yes! Thank you, thank you!" The moment was over, but the power and the love of God had permeated my soul anew.

The day was Tuesday, March 13. A central venous catheter with a long plastic tube was inserted through my chest above the right breast into a main vein. The point of insertion was bandaged and taped. A short plastic tube dangled from my skin and would be a part of me for the next several months. This tube would be the vehicle for the journey of chemo which would soon flow through my body. Now I had two foreign objects in me—one that could lead to my death and one that hopefully would be a pathway to continued life.

As we waited for Dr. Cristofanilli, my knees were weak and my palms were clammy. Waiting, waiting! It is so disconcerting. Imagination runs wild and time seems to stand still. When he entered the examining room, he greeted us with a warm and gentle smile. He uttered the words, "a nasty little tumor," and my anxiety level skyrocketed! He said that it was very aggressive in nature. My mind can't grasp why it hadn't shown on my routine mammogram six months earlier, or why I hadn't felt anything as recently as three months ago. Dave and I were acutely aware that Dr. Cristofanilli was highly concerned as he explained that it was not estrogen-receptive, but urged me to cease taking hormone replacement therapy. He said that while on chemotherapy I should not ingest any vitamins or over-the-counter remedies including aspirin, ibuprofen, and supplements of any kind. He wanted nothing to interfere or intermix with the chemo—such a substance might change the properties of the chemicals. As he spoke, I recall thinking, "Is it really me sitting in this room having this conversation? Is it my body that we are discussing? How strange!"

MD Anderson is a research institution, so there are always trials based on the newest research breakthroughs and expectations. I was asked if I preferred the standard treatment of one week on the taxol chemotherapy with three weeks off for a period of four months (four treatments), or if I would be willing to participate in a newer approach which was taxol each week for three weeks with the fourth week off for the same duration of four months (twelve treatments). We were told that if we agreed to the latter approach, my name would be put into the computer for a random selection of acceptance into the trial. Dave and I both felt that we would like to be a part of the newer research data, and my name was submitted. Within minutes, we were told that I had been accepted and that my first treatment was to be the following morning.

The protocol would be twelve doses of taxol followed by four treatments of a different chemo called FAC, which would be administered in the format of the standard treatment. In October, I would have surgery—either mastectomy or lumpectomy—followed by six weeks of daily radiation Monday through Friday. Before we left that day, Dr. Cristofanilli said that very often the aggressive tumors respond very well to chemo treatments. There was a ray of comfort in that remark, and we thanked him for his efforts and concern on my behalf.

My head was swimming in a sea of information. Couldn't I just bury my head in my pillow and forget about what lay ahead? Luckily, Dave had been so astute with the practicalities of this whole adventure. He remained organized and skillful with the paper work, the questions, and the logistics. He sought information which enhanced our knowledge about my condition. Still, we agreed that our ultimate trust lay in God, in the power of prayer that was being offered on my behalf by so many people, in the expertise of Dr. Cristofanilli and MD Anderson, and in the drugs which have been painstakingly and meticulously researched and then utilized by women who were willing to be involved in experimental trials. To those women who have endured this route before me, I was, and am, humbly grateful.

13

Coincidence? I Think Not!

The phone rang early on the morning of Wednesday, March 14. When I answered, I was warmly greeted by the voice of a man whom I have not seen in over thirty-six years. His name is Joe. He and I shared a very special relationship during our college years in the early 60's in Potsdam, New York. We knew then that we would always have a tender place in our hearts for each other, but that a long-term commitment would never happen. When I graduated in January of 1965, I married Dave, my high school sweetheart, who had been part of my life since I was sixteen years old. Joe and I lost touch.

As the years went by, I continued to wonder what had happened to Joe. My dear friend Mary Ellen, who also graduated from Potsdam, but whom I never met until the late 70's, knew about my curiosity as to Joe's whereabouts. A month before I found the breast cancer, Mary Ellen found Joe's e-mail address on the Internet. I asked Dave if he minded if I sent Joe an e-mail, and he just said, "Go for it!" So I did.

Joe called soon after receiving my e-mail and we had a wonderful conversation reminiscing and catching up on each other's lives. His career, among other things, included knowledge of pharmaceuticals and drugs. He said he would call again in a few weeks.

And so on the morning that I was to begin chemotherapy, I was greeted by his voice. His first question was, "What have you been up to these past couple of months since we last spoke?" I told him that I had been diagnosed with cancer. His deep and troubled concern touched my heart. He immediately asked about the protocol, and I told him that I was to begin chemotherapy in just a few hours with a drug called taxol. He said, "Oh, Sue, taxol is a great drug!" Those words from my long-lost friend were music to my ears. I could hardly wait to get started. Before Joe hung up, he told me that he attended daily Mass at his church and that he would pray for me every day.

Was it coincidence that Joe was reintroduced into my life after thirty-six years? I don't think so! God had simply and powerfully given me yet another gift to aid in my battle—the assurance that Joe could offer me regarding the taxol, and his daily intercessory prayers on my behalf. How incredibly blessed I felt that morning.

On the way to MD Anderson, on this fourteenth day of March, which was the anniversary of my beloved grandmother's birthday, Dave asked if I was nervous. I smiled and said with great confidence, "Today is the day the physical battle against this intrusive monster in my body will begin. I'm ready. Let's go!"

14

The Drip of the Fluids Mirrored My Heartbeat

Dave and I were led into a small, private room in the chemo area by a wonderfully sweet and kind nurse. The room had a comfortable bed, a chair, a television, a cabinet with supplies, and an IV pole. We made ourselves at home and both of us were relieved that our surroundings were so pleasant. The nurse offered me a heated blanket, and I lay down on the bed allowing the warmth of the cover to envelop me as I acclimated myself to this procedure. So strange to think that it would become so familiar and reassuring and comforting over the next several months! In the silence I could hear other patients talking, laughing, crying, or suffering through dry heaves. I simply didn't know what to expect, but I was ready and I sensed calmness within my soul. I closed my eyes and praised God for his presence and his incredible love for me. Dave set the television on an easy-listening music channel which also displayed beautiful pictures of colorful and awesome creations of God. I was truly at peace.

The nurse returned and told us that my blood work indicated I was good to go. She gave me oral antinausea medication, then hooked up the bags of liquid to the IV pole and attached them to the catheter in my chest. The three liquids were Benadryl, a steroid, and the taxol. For the next several hours, I lay on the bed and watched first the Benadryl, then the steroid, and then the taxol slowly and steadily drip, drip, drip on their journey through the plastic tube into the catheter and into my body. The drip of the fluids mirrored my heartbeat, and I took great comfort in the knowledge that with each breath I took and with each beat of my heart, the drip, drip, drip of that precious liquid was the healing potion that would save my life. The Benadryl made me a little sleepy and occasionally I dozed. But when a complete lunch including soup, sandwich, chips, an apple, yogurt, juice, and *two* cookies was brought to me, I ate. I did share *some* with

Dave, but the big joke around my family is that Sue never misses her three square meals a day. So why should this day be any different?

****

I sensed calmness within my soul.

****

Oh, how grateful I was for this first encounter with chemo! I didn't know how I would feel in a few hours, or tomorrow, or later in the week, but right then I felt better than I had in weeks. My spirits were lifted as I sensed the battle initiate between the ugly cancer cells and the beautiful drug. Oh, how I was cheering for the beautiful drug to be the winner. Go taxol! Go taxol!

Dave and I laughed, cried, and praised God for such a glorious day. After dinner (which, of course, I ate), Mike called and almost sheepishly asked how I was feeling. I told him that I had experienced a wonderful day, and that I had just eaten a pork chop, applesauce, broccoli, and rice. There was such relief in his voice as he explained that he could hardly stay focused at work all day just imagining me "holding the toilet bowl." I so loved his precious concern! In the dark of night, I prayed for patients everywhere who are enduring this dreaded disease and suffering from extensive nausea and vomiting while being treated with the powerful chemotherapy drugs. And I thanked God that at least in my initial treatment, I had escaped that misery.

15

Is Bald Really Beautiful?

With the onset of the chemo treatments came the realization that very soon I would lose my hair. For women, the thought of being bald can bring an eeriness of horror and cold sweats as we try to perceive life without our hair, which vanity has allowed to partially define who we are. A bald man can have a look of virility and sex appeal which can actually enhance his looks and masculinity, but that's not true for most women. I admire the women whose self-confidence and courage have set them free to be themselves in their own baldness. But for most of us, hair is such an integral part of our feminine being that I know some even refuse chemo treatments because they do not want to lose what their hair represents. How we perceive our own individual looks is so completely tied into our ego, our self-esteem, our feminine appeal, and our vanity. Whew! I wondered how I would respond to the reality of baldness when it ultimately invades my world.

I had been blessed with thick, coarse, manageable hair which had been a lush shade of auburn in my younger days. But since I ceased coloring it several months before the cancer reared its ugly head, I was currently sporting a mane of pure white. Decisions, decisions! Should I purchase a wig with the chic white look of today, or should I return to the medium blonde hue of a year ago? Or should I completely relinquish my inhibitions and brave the alluring reddish look of my youth?

****
… hair is such an integral part of our feminine being ….
****

Dave and I visited three shops and shared many a laugh over the way I looked in some of the weird and exotic wigs available. In the end, my conservative nature defeated the wild streak of my imagination and I chose a wig that reminded me of my own hair over the better part of the past twenty years. Yet I only wore it eight or ten times. I much preferred the colorful biker scarves and fun, perky hats which would soon become part of my everyday wardrobe.

It was kind of fun picking out a new, fashionable look for my head. Yet I found it strange that I and the other women shopping for what would hide our baldness from the world and perhaps even from ourselves were so cordial and upbeat and complimentary to one another! "Oh, I love that color on you;" "Now that one is so youthful and perky-looking;" "Oh, that one really brings out the blue in your eyes;" "You look great in that one;" "Maybe you should get them both!"

Instead of the pleasantries, why weren't we all crying and yelling and tearing our hair out? After all, it wouldn't be long before it would be falling out on its own anyway. My God, we were in the clutches of cancer! We were each desperately trying to face the realization that life had maliciously inflicted this vicious disease on us. But instead of that inner turmoil, what I saw was the inner strength, the ability to cope, the faith, the hope, the need to function, the capacity to overcome, the brave attempt to make lemonade out of this lemon we all shared as we strolled around the wig shops and cancer boutiques. Fate had brought us here. But it was the need for normalcy amidst the anguish, for peace and serenity and compassion amidst the fears that held us captive, for the laughter and gentleness and grace amidst the flow of tears and uncertainty, which kept each of us sane and productive and hopeful.

An elementary school friend of mine with whom I'd had little communication over the years called me when she heard of my illness and said, "Don't hide under the covers, but rather get up each morning and put one foot in front of the other all day long." What sage advice! That became my motto.

16

My Daily Routine

My days were filled with routine, with joyous reminders of life and love, with incredible awareness of my own body, with emotions that vacillated between the high road and the low, with intense desire to stay in God's presence through prayer and scripture.

My daily routine began in the early morning. I was up by 7:30 no matter how many hours of sleep I had enjoyed the previous night. My sleep patterns were terribly irregular. Some nights I felt blessed to get even four or five hours. I began to take Ambien 5 mg several nights a week. Sometimes it helped. But mostly, the nighttime demons kept me awake. And since I had been taken off hormone replacement therapy, my friend Jo reminded me that I was probably again enduring the "joys" of menopause. Oh, great!

Each morning I injected a vial of Heprin into the catheter in my chest in order to keep the line open and clean. Because of the port which was taped to my chest, I found early on that the shower was too nerve-racking. I was so fearful that the bandage would get wet and lead to infection. So I chose to sponge-bathe my upper body at the sink and then lower myself into a warm tub of soothing water to complete the cleansing process. Within the first few days there was no longer a need for shampoo. I simply soaped my head along with my face. That wasn't all bad. It meant there was no more need for a blow-dryer and no more bad hair days. My mouth required three good cleanings each day, which included brushing, flossing, and gargling with salt water. This routine was to help prevent mouth sores, which can be a very uncomfortable side effect of chemo.

I drank eighty to a hundred ounces of water each day to keep my system hydrated and flushed—which of course meant many scurrying trips to the bathroom. I took my temperature regularly, as any fever was to be reported to the doctor. I ate very nutritiously, including extensive servings of green, red, and orange vegetables; red meat; and even liver (ugh!) for iron.

My mother *loved* liver and bacon and onions, so as children we were "treated" to this entrée every month. I *hated* liver—I managed to swallow small pieces by consuming much liquid and feasting on the bacon. What should I do now that liver was being promoted to help my red blood counts? I decided that I wasn't going to cook it but would go to a restaurant instead.

I remembered a time in my mother's later years when dementia ruled her mind. She and Dad had come to Houston for a visit. Dave and I entertained them at a couple of very fine restaurants and I cooked a few gourmet dinners. But one night I took them to Luby's Cafeteria, where she ordered liver and onions and raved about how delicious her meal was. So much for my culinary achievements!

But now that I was advised to tempt my palate with liver, I decided to go to Mom's favorite place. The first time (and there were only three), I sat at the table all by myself, like a little kid really not wanting to expose my mouth and my taste buds to this "thing" on my plate. I concentrated on the onions and mashed potatoes. Finally I took a piece of liver and then another. I found that if I dipped the liver into the potatoes, I didn't gag so much. But after three consecutive weeks, I said to myself, "No more!" I switched to liverwurst sandwiches and smugly congratulated myself that I had found a way to enjoy the benefits of liver without the much dreaded agony of "the real stuff."

I tried to walk at least two miles four days a week, either enjoying the beautiful spring weather or staying inside on my treadmill. Some days I would lie quietly on my bed and listen to a meditative tape for peace and relaxation. I did my chores. I ran my errands. Life went on! I found that my power of concentration failed when I tried to read a book. My mind wandered in every direction and I read the same paragraph over and over.

So I watched old sitcoms—especially in the middle of the night when my mind wouldn't let me sleep. I became reacquainted with the Cosbys and the Jeffersons and Archie and Edith Bunker. Most of the episodes made me laugh. Laughter is so important when dealing with stress. I became obsessed with jigsaw puzzles and crossword puzzles. I also found that as the days and weeks of chemo treatment progressed, I seemed to lose confidence in my own decisions and in my ability to feel independent. My short-term memory seemed less trustworthy. I relied more on Dave, and that was not my normal modus operandi. I moved into the guest room so that I didn't interrupt Dave with my erratic sleep patterns and he didn't disturb me with his gentle snoring (ha ha!) and trips to the bathroom.

Amidst the ho-hum of the routine, I found incredible joy. The outpouring of love, concern, and good wishes was overwhelming to both Dave and me. There were so many e-mails and phone calls and beautiful cards that I cherished and read over and over. I knew that people all over the world were praying for me and I was humbled by that knowledge. Flowers arrived, neighbors brought home-made soup every other week, and people from our Sunday school class delivered delicious dinners. Friends visited. Sometimes we would go out for lunch. Hats arrived as gifts. And when my darling grandson, Jake, would run into my arms, my heart would burst with thanksgiving and excitement and love. One evening on the phone he called me "Ma Ma" for the first time, and my heart exploded with joy! Jake and I have a very special bond, as I had had the privilege of caring for him five days a week until he was eight months old—a time in my life that I cherish deeply.

I became so totally aware of every nuance of my body. What had been just a routine ache, pain, discomfort, or irregularity I now questioned extensively and found myself going to a variety of doctors to be diagnosed and treated. For me, the unknown is what produces the fear. I had grown fairly comfortable with the fact that I was a cancer patient in treatment. But my anxieties over the rest of my symptoms raged uncontrollably.

It seemed that as one problem was eliminated, another would appear so that I experienced continual frustration and concern. A mildly red throat which had been annoying me for weeks before the onset of the cancer journey became con-cern that I could have throat cancer. I didn't. The vertigo which I have experi-enced periodically over the years became a fright that it could be a brain tumor. It wasn't. The pain I had been experiencing in both elbows for several months along with total numbness in my arms when I slept prompted thoughts that my ner-vous system was awry. It wasn't. Severe indigestion and a pain in the center of my chest which lasted for several weeks took me to a gastroenterologist. After an endoscope procedure, I thankfully received a diagnosis of GERD and not stom-ach or esophageal cancer. A brief bout with rectal bleeding prompted a colonos-copy—which I was due to have at my age anyway. The results were perfect. The dentist checked my mouth; the dermatologist scanned my skin. I had had a skin cancer removed from my face four months before the breast lump was found, so I was especially watchful for any further skin abnormalities!

****
There were times when I felt so totally alone.
****

I spent a great deal of time and energy focused on my physical being. Some-times this concentration stole from me my need and desire to focus on God. There were times when I felt a terrible sense of distance from God. I simply could not feel his presence. There were times when I felt so totally alone. But because of my faith, I know deep in my soul that God never leaves us; it is we who leave him. So even when I wasn't feeling the proximity of God, I continued to praise him, to worship him, to read scripture, and to pray to him with thanksgiving for forgiveness and strength and healing.

One particular Sunday when I didn't go to church, I sat by myself in my bedroom with an old hymnal and sang to God, with only the walls to hear. "Holy, Holy, Holy," "How Great Thou Art," "Amazing Grace," and "Here I Am, Lord!" In the solitude of my own room with tears streaming down my face, I knew that God and I were sharing the same space.

17

Who Was Marietta?

My friend Ronnie and I shared many conversations over the weeks and months as we compared notes on our treatments and progress. She prepared me for the possibilities of what might happen next. We continued to laugh through the struggles as we joked about every aspect of our lives and physical conditions. She encouraged me to have my head shaved as soon as my hair started to "fall onto my dinner plate" or "leave its calling card in clumps on my pillow."

After my second chemo treatment on March 21, I began to notice my hair disappearing from all parts of my body. I had only given thought to the hair on my head, but indeed my eyelashes, eyebrows, and even my nose hairs were soon beginning to disappear. The good news was that for several months I didn't have to shave my arms or legs. And think of all the money I saved on razors and shampoo and mousse and hair spray!

By the last week of March, the hair on my head was quite easy to pull out. Although none of it ever left a calling card on my pillow or fell on my dinner plate, I knew it was time. I made an appointment at the beauty salon at MD Anderson to have my head shaved on the morning of March 30. The previous evening, Dave and I had watched the movie *South Pacific* on television, and I sang every song with much gusto and pleasure. But when Mitzi Gaynor sang, "I'm Gonna Wash That Man Right Outta My Hair," the gusto gave way to gentle tears as I accepted the reality that in less than fourteen hours I wouldn't have any hair to wash.

As I sat down in the chair, the very kind woman who was to shave my head turned the chair so that I was facing away from the mirror. Instead, I looked into the face of a lovely young woman, a patient like me, dressed in a white nightgown and robe. The buzz of the electric shaver droned in the quiet stillness of the air.

****

Who was she and why was she in my path on this particular morning?

****

The patient, whose name was Marietta, quietly told me about her own horrendous cancer journey, which included a late-stage tumor, a three-year battle with chemo and radiation, multiple surgeries, a husband who divorced her in the interim, and a God who protected her and loved her and carried her through each and every step. I was enthralled by her joy and her faith and the glow on her face. I was hardly aware of what was happening to me. Who was she and why was she in my path on this particular morning?

Suddenly she said, "Your head is shaped so perfectly, and you look so beautiful!" The buzzing had stopped and I knew that the moment had come. I asked Marietta if I should turn now and look at myself. She smiled and nodded her head.

As I stared at myself in the mirror there was initial shock. I could feel my throat tighten as I choked back the tears. I thought about Marietta's words of comfort when she said that I looked beautiful. I thought about myself as a person not defined by my outer appearance. With thumbs up, I smiled and turned to Dave to acknowledge my baldness. I saw tears cascading down his face. I knew that he was feeling a deep empathy for me. He smiled and returned my gesture—two thumbs up. I tied one of my chic biker scarves around my head and stated that I thought I looked really cute. Dave and I laughed and hugged, and Marietta was gone. Funny, I never saw her leave the room, and she never said good-bye. Was she my guardian angel? I told Dave that I thought God had given me the gift of Marietta to encourage me and help me through that dreaded moment, letting me know again that he was with me and would never forsake me on my journey through cancer or through life.

When we arrived home, I stood in front of the mirror looking at my baldness for a very long time. I indulged in a small pity party and cried as I understood that, whether left au natural in its baldness or covered in my recently acquired head attire, this new look was the outward manifestation of the reality of my illness. Up until that moment, my physical being hadn't been noticeably changed, but now it would be clear to the world that I was a cancer statistic.

Jim arrived in the afternoon and asked to see my head. I was hesitant, and I'm not sure if that was for his sake or for mine. But he was insistent, so I removed the scarf. Jim simply smiled, rubbed his hands gently over my hairless head, and said I looked cool. I was so relieved. I quietly cried, and we held each other in silence and in love.

That evening I sat at Enron Field (now known as Minute Maid Park) to watch my beloved Astros play baseball. I was surrounded by my entire family as we celebrated my fifty-eighth birthday on April 1. We were doing what I enjoy so much—cheering the Astros. Mike, Marla, and Jake had met us there and gave me such big hugs and tender comments about my "new do in the biker scarf." If only I'd had a Harley, I'd have been *really* cool. The roof of the park was open, the stars were shining, the breeze was cool and refreshing, my family was together having fun, and the Astros won.

It doesn't get much better than that. Thank you, God!

18

Excerpts from My Journal—April 2001

Sunday, April 1

Today I am fifty-eight! Another milestone in this journey on earth called life! What is life but a gift from God? Each day, no matter our circumstances, we can choose to walk the path which will glorify our creator by being obedient, by being humble, by being grateful, by being kind and loving and compassionate, by praising God! Some days that journey seems monumentally difficult, but today my heart swells with joy and I thank God that I am fifty-eight, and that I am his!

Thursday, April 5

The sun is shining in all of its brilliance, the sky is a deep blue, the billowy white clouds race across the heavens, and the glory of God surrounds Dave and me as we meander our way through the hill country of Texas. It is a perfect day of rest in the beautiful countryside as we oooh and aaah at the spectacular fields of blue-bonnets and other glorious multi-colored wild flowers. It is easy to get lost in the splendor of God's creation and in his power amidst such beauty and peace.

Saturday, April 7

The strong and purposeful commentary of my Scripture reading today (James 1:19, 20) admonishes one to "be angry at the injustices of the world, but not to be angry because our personal feelings have been hurt!" Wow! A light bulb flashes in my head as I realize how much time and energy I have spent being angry at the personal hurts that I perceive have been inflicted on me, particularly by Dave, over the years of my life. The Bible continues by saying that the responsive anger and retaliatory behavior which I exhibit because of these personal hurt feelings is a great sin. It's like saying, "Two wrongs don't make a right." Believe it or not, this is a wonderful revelation! It's not about me! It's about acting in a way that is pleasing to God! Our culture and the world around us so often generate the concept that life should center solely on what is pleasing to us! And the disappointments follow in abundance because that is not the purpose of our being. We are here to glorify God and seek his will for justice in a world that is deeply distressed and in need of our prayers and concerns and action. Whew! I am excited and relieved. I ask God to forgive me and then go to Dave and apologize for my ungodly attitudes and actions in dealing with my own personal hurt feelings.

Monday, April 9

Isn't dealing with all of the ramifications of breast cancer enough? I was overcome today with the anxiety of my physical condition. I couldn't seem to control the sobs which wracked my body! My emotions evoked pity as I dealt with the anger I was feeling at being subjected to so many "little annoyances and ailments" both related to and unrelated to the cancer treatment. Like King David in the Psalms, I cried out to God for his comfort and his guidance in helping me to find resolution and peace!

Tuesday, April 10

Dave and I went to the movies today. My concentration was less than desired when suddenly I had the most urgent sense of panic. I wanted to run away! I envisioned myself moving out of my physical body and leaving the dreadful cancer behind. But the reality is that I cannot escape. I am trapped with this disease like a prisoner. I am not free to run away for there is nowhere that I can go that the cancer will not be there also. It reminded me of how many people live their lives "incarcerated" due to their life circumstances. My Uncle Ben survived the tortures, starvation, and duress of being a prisoner of war during World War II. Others are imprisoned by fear, oppression, bitterness, materialism, greed, loneliness, poverty, disease. While the movie continued, I prayed for people everywhere who are trapped by the human condition. And as the tears spilled slowly down my face, my panic subsided. For although the world is not always a pretty place, I find comfort in knowing that God walks with us even as he weeps for our individual and collective plights!

Thursday, April 12

I was standing at the window across from the chemo area waiting to be escorted to my room to receive the drip, drip, drip of the wondrous drugs which would soon roam through my body attacking the nasty cancer cells. I was joyously and humbly thanking and praising God for the wonderful news that Dave and I had just received from Dr. Cristofanilli. He said that the tumor had softened and flattened and was palpable. He also said the nodes under my arm had shrunk, and that a questionable node in my neck area was confirmed as benign. The taxol and the prayers were working!

As I turned to go into the waiting area, I came face-to-face with a woman who was smiling at me. She was dressed in the garb of an MD Anderson maintenance person, and we later found out that her name was Ida and that she cleaned the chemo rooms. She warmly took my hand and said that as she was pushing her cleaning cart past the waiting area, the Lord spoke to her and said, "Go to the woman at the window and tell her to be encouraged in the Lord!" I was simply astonished! I could hardly believe my ears! I took both of her hands and then hugged her. Half-laughing and half-crying, I thanked her profusely for delivering such a profound message. She said that she would pray for me, and then she left to fulfill her earthly duties. Dave and I couldn't keep from smiling at another unexpected and incredible gift from God. But what impressed us the most was the fact that when Ida heard God speak to her, she was obedient to his call. How I pray to be such a faithful servant!

That evening when we returned home from our day at the hospital buoyed by the good news from the doctor and from Ida, there was a card in the mail from our son Mike, telling me that he loves me and is thinking about me. How beautiful is *that* special gift from God?

Thursday–Sunday, April 12–15

Holy Week always creates in me a deep humility and a powerful yearning to grow closer to Jesus. I am moved to tears by the music and the prayers and The Word elicited from the various church services on Maundy Thursday, Good Friday, and Easter Sunday. This week I reflect on the prayer of Jabez (1 Chronicles 4:10). A servant of God, he prays that God might bless him, indeed, and enlarge his territory—that God would give him his hand and keep him from evil so that he might not endure or cause anyone pain! What a bold and entreating and humbling prayer! I like that! My regret is that neither Dave nor I had pursued God and discovered a relationship with Jesus on a daily journey earlier in our lives. Perhaps had we done that, our family life would have been God-focused and we wouldn't have caused each other and our children so much pain.

Now I love the sense of being in God's presence knowing that he knows me—the good, the bad, and the ugly—and yet loves me incomprehensibly in spite of myself. As I partake of the Holy Communion, I bow my head in reverence with deepest thanksgiving for the pain and misery which Jesus endured, so that I might be forgiven and saved to live eternally with God. *That* is the greatest gift of all!

Tuesday, April 17

While I was talking on the phone to my friend Kim, who always seems to know exactly when I need a little cheering up, I was aware that the yard man was peering at me through the window with a very quizzical look on his face. Three or four times, he seemingly did double-takes as I glanced in his direction. Finally I looked down at my clothes to see if something was askew, and then I went to the mirror to see if I was wearing my breakfast on my face. I started to laugh. The poor man was probably trying to figure out if I was male or female as I was dressed in jeans and a very baggy sweatshirt with no head covering. My bald head was standing out like a sore thumb. So I feminized myself with lipstick and a pretty head scarf and casually wandered over to the window. He smiled looking very relieved to have his problem solved. I am sure that he had a great time telling his friends about the strange "lady" with the bald head.

Thursday, April 19

Today I received my fifth chemo treatment. Hooray—only eleven more to go! I am amazed how routine and natural it all seems. My blood counts today were great; my immune system is holding really well. I feel wonderful. Before the chemo treatment, I went, as I do each week, to have the dressing changed at the port site on my chest. No infection, no damaged skin from the tape. I am humbled and grateful at how fortunate I am as I plod along on this journey. Over the past few days I have noticed weakness in my hands (harder to open jars), and a sense of burning and tingling in my fingers and toes. Is that from the taxol? I am aware that neuropathy is a potential side effect of the drug. I am wide awake tonight, as usually happens after chemo because of the steroid drip which precedes the taxol. I wonder if the gift of sleep will come tonight. Oh, well, there's always the jigsaw puzzle or "Nick at Nite" on television to keep me company.

Saturday, April 21

What a beautiful wedding! I am here in Florida surrounded by my own family and the extended Teall family to witness the marriage of our beautiful niece Wendy and her sweetheart, Aaron. I pray for this young couple—as they begin their journey as husband and wife—to always focus on God first in their lives, and then on each other. The newlyweds are replaced in my mind by our son Mike and his wife, Marla, for whom I offer the same prayer. I reach for Dave's hand and we share a squeeze and a smile. We are both so well aware of how much we really do love each other "for better or worse, for richer or poorer, in sickness and in health."

In the parking lot of the hotel, Dave and I were walking to our room after the wedding festivities had ended. I was complaining about how hot and uncomfortable I felt in my wig. He simply reached over, yanked the wig off of my head and began twirling it in his hand. I looked up to see people standing on their room balcony looking rather shocked in their disbelief as we laughed our way into the lobby.

I am tired, but overjoyed with such a special day of love and family.

Monday, April 23

Weepy farewells, lots of hugs, and much encouragement came from Dave's family as we all headed home in different directions. I am so glad that I overcame my hesitancy and fear of leaving the security of being in Houston near my doctor, and instead ventured to Florida for this wonderful event and supportive family reunion.

We enjoyed the last few hours with my Aunt Audrey and Uncle Ben, who journeyed from their home in Florida to spend precious time with Dave and me, Jim, Mike, Marla, and our darling little Jake. As I was prancing around au natural, my uncle kept calling me "Telly," as in Telly Savalas who starred in a television show called *Kojak* many years ago. Kojak had a beautiful bald head, continually sucked small lollipops, and his trademark line was, "Who loves ya, baby?" Ben and Audrey had brought me a huge box of lollipops so that I could adopt the persona of Kojak and greet people with a lollipop dangling from my lips saying, "Who loves ya, baby?" What fun and laughter!

As we shared a tear bidding them farewell, I hugged my aunt and thanked her for her humorous, upbeat, encouraging support—and for the many hats she had sent over the past weeks.

(Little did I know at the time I wrote this entry into my journal, that this farewell would literally be the final one. I never saw her again as she died December 19, 2001, from postsurgical complications while I was still journeying through my cancer struggle in daily radiation treatments.)

Friday, April 27

Today I had an ultrasound. Isn't it strange how we focus our eyes on the face of the technician hoping for any expression that will tell us what we want to hear? About fifteen minutes after the test was complete, time I spent alone in the sterility of the testing room in earnest prayer and wary anticipation, the radiologist made a grand entrance into the examining room with the words, "Well, God damn, the tumor is barely there!" After the momentary shock of the way the test results were presented, my emotions took over and the tears, which constantly lie in wait ever so close to the spillover point, found their way onto my cheeks. How am I supposed to feel? My emotions are all over the map. I want to shout with joy, but I don't want to jump the gun on expectation. I am humbled and thankful, but I know there is a huge journey still ahead. Will this news change the protocol of my treatment? What *is* my future? I am excited, I am cautious, I am weepy.

Dave hears the news and is similarly tentative in his reaction, but as we leave the building, he grabs my hand and starts shouting, "Whoopee, whoopee, whoopee!" Maybe it's okay to celebrate and jump for joy for this precious moment in time which has given us so much hope! I smile as I close my eyes tonight, thanking God for the incredible gift of hope.

19

God's Special Gifts

Dave and I were patiently sitting in the waiting area of the Breast Clinic at MD Anderson anticipating my May appointment with Dr. Cristofanilli. The area seemed more crowded than usual, and we soon learned that the doctor was not only seeing his own patients, but filling in for another doctor due to an emergency. We hunkered down in our seats, knowing that the wait would be even longer than usual. I remember thinking about the dedication and long hours that this incredible staff endures while dealing with patient after patient suffering from this hideous disease. The doctors at MD Anderson not only see patients during the practical, human application of their profession, but spend countless hours a week doing research to continually learn more about the disease and potential treatments. Why? What drives them? What led them to this intense vocation which involves so much suffering and pain and death? I cannot imagine myself working in such an occupation.

I marvel at God's plan for humanity. Unlike the other creatures which roam the earth, men and women are given spiritual gifts, skills, talents, desires, and free will to make choices in their lives. Innately, we are all gifted by God with different attributes and intellects and uniqueness that allow for choices of great variance and numerous possibilities. None of us can totally comprehend the reasoning for each personal choice nor the vast amount of data needed to be understood in order to be proficient in any given choice. How exciting that God has gifted each of us in such a way that the possibilities in life are endless!

****

I marvel at God's plan for humanity.

****

However, society and cultural environments do not always allow these gifts to develop and flourish. Sadly, whole groups of people are stifled by circumstances out of their control, such as oppression, war, extreme poverty, and epidemic conditions. Some of us do not ever pursue or even recognize our gifts, so we don't utilize them to the fullest, or we abuse them recklessly by being enticed into the darkness of temptation and wrong doing. Nevertheless, I believe that God does have a unique journey for each of us. It is our duty to determine what that journey is, and then proceed to the best of our God-given abilities within the circumstances of our lives—perhaps even rising above and foiling the circumstances.

It was after 4:30 when Dr. Cristofanilli walked into the examination room. He greeted us with his usual smile and gracious manner, but he looked so very exhausted. After he physically checked me, he said, "Let me take a look at the reports from the radiologist in regards to the ultrasound." Of course Dave and I already had heard the results from the radiologist a couple of weeks prior when I was told that after six taxol treatments, the tumor was eighty-four percent gone.

Suddenly, Dr. Cristofanilli's entire demeanor changed from exhaustion to elation as he was practically shouting, "This is amazing! Wow! This is the best possible news!" We experienced a sense of pure joy as we witnessed him relish the news that, at that precise moment in time, in my particular body, all of his efforts and those of his dedicated cohorts working in the field of breast cancer were being rewarded. He was genuinely uplifted in his own spirit and so very excited and hopeful for me. We shared a hug, and I had an inkling of why he is so devoted to his patients and to furthering the research which will one day render breast cancer obsolete. Thank you, God, for Dr. Cristofanilli and his colleagues, who are using their God-given talents and gifts for the benefit of humanity.

20

What Is Happening to Me?

I have usually been able to handle difficult circumstances and make decisions rather confidently throughout my life. I recall a time when we were living in Anacortes, Washington. Dave was involved in labor negotiations at work and was actually "locked in" on the premises as the contract deadline drew near.

One morning a toilet in our home on the lower level overflowed, which was certainly not adding to my day. I knew not to bother Dave at work with such trivia. I remembered that, the preceding day, the utility company had installed a street light on our front property, so I determined that they must have done something which was now causing my current situation. When I called the company, I was told that they would come out with a backhoe and dig up a portion of our front yard to determine if they were responsible, but that I would have a rather large bill to pay if they had not been negligent. I was so confident in my reasoning that I told the company employee to proceed with the big dig.

I must admit to a tad of nervous tension as I watched my yard being dismantled, but the result proved that the utility company was indeed responsible for crushing a portion of our sewer line, thus causing my toilet to overflow. After releasing my long-held breath, I allowed myself to relax with a deep sigh of relief. When Dave arrived home a couple of days later, he was flabbergasted at what I had done. I know that he was picturing the dollar signs had I been wrong. But as he turned away, I saw just the hint of a smile cross his face. He knew that I "had done good!"

****

Sometimes I felt confused ....
****

That is why, as I proceeded further into the taxol treatments, I was dumbfounded at my seeming inability to make decisions, my lack of self-confidence and my anxiety when Dave was not close by. For example, I love to drive and prefer to be at the wheel rather than to be a passenger. But I began to actually be relieved when Dave was doing the driving. How could that be? Sometimes I felt confused, and my memory seemed to be failing me at times.

I knew Dave's fishing trip was fast approaching. He's been fishing biannually with the same twelve men for over twenty-five years, and he always looks forward to the fun and the fishing and the camaraderie. Deep down, although he was only going to be away for four nights about two hundred and fifty miles from home, I was anxious about being alone and didn't really want him to go. I never expressed this to anyone, especially Dave, because I saw myself as a wimp and was embarrassed to admit that I was afraid! And the ironic part was that I really did not know what the culprit was that was responsible for my fear!

Lo and behold, a few days before he was to leave, my dear friend, Paulette, whose husband is one of the esteemed fishermen, called and said that she was coming to Houston for a few days while the gang fished and that she would love to stay with me. I all but shrieked with delight and relief! We had wonderful quality time together. She is such a woman of faith whom I admire, and we shared deeply about so much! She brought me a bag full of seven gifts to be opened each day for a week after she left. What a treasure—a gift each day with a special card and spiritual message or biblical verse! But more than those gifts, the genuinely true treasure was the gift of Paulette, whom God had brought to me when I needed her most!

21

Who Says I Can't Remember?

I have been very competitive all of my life. Most times my spirit of competitiveness is for the love of the sport or the game. I honestly feel that I am a good loser as well as a good winner. But deep down, I usually do want to win. Even if I am just walking around the indoor track at the Y, I want to pass the person in front of me, or at least better my own personal time. (The exception is my genuine hope that my grandson will legitimately beat me at Sorry or Bingo or the like, which he often does.)

So when MD Anderson asked if I would participate in a memory test being given to taxol patients (one of the several study protocols in which I participated), I readily agreed. Although I perceived that I had been experiencing a diminished ability in my short-term memory, I was determined to ace that test. The test comprised a series of words which I either heard from the instructor or saw on a piece of paper, which I then had to recollect in a timed effort. The degree of difficulty increased with each segment. I also had to remember patterns which I had been shown and then reconstruct them with pegs. I knew that the test was going to command my undivided attention and absolute concentration. But there was no way that this test was going to defeat me!

When the test was completed, the instructor, who sensed my eagerness and seriousness, just shook her head in laughter. "You must be pretty competitive," she said. "You just blew the top off this test. No one who has taken it so far has scored anywhere close to your score!"

"Yeah!" I said to myself. "I did it!"

When I arrived home that evening, Dave asked me the name of the instructor and I couldn't remember. But I had aced the test!

22

Facing My Own Death

It was the middle of the night, perhaps around 3:00 AM. I was awakened by the ferocious sounds of thunder and the flashes of lightening which produced eerie images around the guest room where I was supposed to be slumbering. The world outside my window was agitated and restless and in an intense uproar. I lay there in the security of my bed for many moments, reconciling myself to the storminess outside my window, when I suddenly felt myself in that same state of torment. I began to cry in desperation, telling God over and over that I did not want to die! I was frantic and seemingly out of control! And that was strange because I never really did think that I would die from the cancer which I had already been told was disappearing from my body. What was happening to me? Why was I suddenly so paranoid about my own death?

As the thunder and the lightening began to subside in the dark of the night, a glorious sensation invaded my mind and my body. I knew that the violence of my emotional outcry to God just moments before was the outpouring of my unresolved fear of death. I knew that it was at that precise moment, when I was so vulnerable in my fear, that God clearly and without any doubt revealed his assurance to me that I was right with him. I no longer have to fear my own death whenever that time comes. For my inner soul and God's will are entwined. In that moment, I understood the promise of my eternal salvation with Christ so strongly that my body and my mind succumbed to an incredible relaxation and peace. I praise God for this revelation and I rest in his promise. What a sense of relief to be so certain of my future!

23

God Speaks to His Children

I was talking on the phone with Ronnie, my breast cancer patient friend in Florida. We were, as usual, comparing notes, laughing, encouraging one another, sharing stories, and boosting each other's egos. She was describing her surgery as I listened intently. It was time for me to begin to consider the surgical options afforded me by my particular situation. What would be best? What would induce the desired results for continued survival? Should I just be rid of the diseased breast, or should I have both removed in hopes that I would feel less fearful that the disease might occur in the right breast? I knew that MD Anderson's philosophy was to try to preserve the breast if at all possible. Therefore, was a lumpectomy a viable alternative?

As Ronnie and I were saying our farewells and wishing each other a good week ahead, another call was coming through. When I switched to the second call, a recorded voice said, "This is not a sales call. Do you know that you have been healed by God?" The female voice then quoted five or six scripture readings about healing. I was so dumbfounded that I could not process what Bible verses she was reiterating. I sank into my chair. I could simply not fathom what was happening! And then she was gone. Who was this? And why was I the recipient of the message? I was stunned, but as I sat there in the quiet of my room, I began to reflect on all of the different and special and unique ways in which God had communicated with me over these past months. Could it be? Was it really? I smiled to myself, bowed my head and simply said, "Thank you!" And somehow I knew that God was smiling, too.

24

Life Just Isn't Fair

In the span of about thirty minutes, my heart, which had felt like a balloon ready to burst with pride inside my chest, suddenly ached with compassion and sadness!

Our son, Jim, was completing his tenure at Memorial Drive Presbyterian Church as Director of the Young Singles program. Soon he would leave to begin a new staff position at First Presbyterian Church. He invited Dave and me to attend his final evening session with this group of young adults—individuals filled with exuberance, seeking God's will in their lives, loving fun, and sharing troubles. Of course, many of them had been praying for me for several weeks, so it afforded me an opportunity to thank them for their concern and good wishes and fervent prayers. Jim spoke eloquently about new beginnings, friendships, and trusting God. He never ceases to amaze me with the wisdom and depth of understanding of God and of life which he is able to share with his listeners. I was filled with a humble sense of joy.

After the formal part of the evening concluded, Jim introduced me to a young woman in her twenties who was new to the group and who had discovered a lump in her breast. She was frightened, alone, and without insurance. She had been told by a clinic dealing with Medicaid patients that she could get an appointment for a biopsy in three months. My heart broke for her! I tried to encourage her, told her I would pray for her, and asked if she would mind if I called to check on her. She gave me her phone number, we hugged, and then she left. Over the next several days, I left messages on her recorder three or four times, but she never returned my calls. Neither Jim nor I ever saw her again.

****

I do not know why life isn't fair!

****

As I lay in my bed that night, I reflected on the unfairness of life. I was being treated at one of the most prestigious cancer institutions in the world, covered by my husband's company insurance, while this young woman of little economic means was waiting three months for a test which would determine her immediate future. Life surely is not fair!

I remembered the words of a minister in Cancun, Mexico where Dave and I had led a group of sixteen-year-olds, including Jim, on a work project mission trip many years before. The young people were feeling guilty and bewildered by the fact that each of us had so much materially while the Mexican families with whom we were working had so very little. "It just isn't fair," our group clamored! The minister replied, "No, it is not fair, but it is life. Do not feel guilty. None of us can help where we are born and into what circumstances. Your job, as materially blessed Americans, is to go back home, become the best at whatever it is that you choose to become, and then share yourselves and your wealth with the world."

I do not know why life isn't fair! But I do know, thanks to the wisdom of that Mexican minister, that I, who have been given much, have a responsibility to share more of my time, my talents and my resources with the less fortunate around the world. After all, "they" didn't choose the circumstances of their birth any more than I did.

25

The Twenty-Third Psalm

The Twenty-Third Psalm has always spoken to my heart with an eloquence of peace and hope and comfort. It was recited at both of my parents' memorial services, and allowed me to be totally aware of God's assurances in life and in death. From the New International Version Bible, the Psalm is as follows:

The Lord is my shepherd, I shall not be in want.
He makes me lie down in green pastures,
He leads me beside quiet waters,
He restores my soul.
He guides me in paths of righteousness
For his name's sake.
Even though I walk
Through the valley of the shadow of death,
I will fear no evil,
For your rod and your staff,
They comfort me.
You prepare a table before me
In the presence of my enemies,
You anoint my head with oil;
My cup overflows.
Surely goodness and love will follow me
All the days of my life,
And I will dwell in the house of the Lord forever!

Within the very first few days of my diagnosis, I expressed to Dave my desire to have a small card for my wallet, or a bookmark, or a magnet for the refrigerator, on which these poignant words were written. I knew that the proximity of those words would be a continuous reminder and comfort to me of God's amazing love. But for some reason, we never did make that purchase.

One Sunday afternoon, while Jim was at our house, Mike arrived at the door with a wrapped gift under his arm. He simply said, "I hope you like it!" It was a framed print of the Twenty-Third Psalm. Unbeknownst to him, he had given me the words of scripture that I had so much wanted to have close to me. As I looked at him through the mist of my tears, I could see in his eyes the reflection of his soul and his heart. I could see love and forgiveness and fear. Dave and I shared a remorseful, yet hopeful glance with one another. It was a moment in time in which the world seemed to stop! No one spoke. We all knew the significance.

Over the past few years Mike and Jim had both been struggling with the angers, hurts, and residual repercussions in their lives which they felt they were experiencing partly because of childhood insecurities and disappointments resulting from certain parental decisions and behavior patterns. Because of this, there had been periods of estrangement and separation of hearts among all of us. Often when we were together, there was more tension than joy. But through the grace of God, much soul-searching, repentance, forgiveness, and a deep desire for reconciliation on all of our hearts, we are slowly redefining our roles as parents and grandparents, and theirs as adult children. We are concentrating on the present and relishing the future rather than being mired in the past.

I am always amazed and humbled by the manner in which God continually evokes good even when we are faced with the most severe struggles and disappointments and heartaches of our lives. For, at that precious moment when Mike and I shared the Twenty-Third Psalm, we as a family unit were also sharing a peace and a thanksgiving and a love for one another and for God. I am so grateful!

26

The Dreaded Neuropathy Arrives

By the latter part of May, my toes and the balls of my feet were stiff and painful. A burning sensation was a constant source of discomfort. It started in my toes, which were beginning to ooze under the nails, and slowly crawled past my ankles up toward my knees. It felt as if I had been outdoors in subfreezing conditions with my toes numb from the cold and then had put my feet into a bucket of warm water. Anyone who has experienced that sensation knows exactly what I mean.

Shoes were becoming impossible to wear because of the intolerable discomfort, so I spent many weeks in one pair of open-toed sandals which were the most bearable. The good news was that I never had to waste time making a decision about what to wear on my feet. (Those shoes quickly found the trash bin when all was said and done.) Keeping my feet in a propped position seemed to offer some relief, so I ungraciously usurped Dave's comfy recliner in the den as my own chair. He was more than willing to relinquish his favorite spot to my miserable feet.

****

This cancer business is definitely not for the faint of heart!
****

My hands and fingers were also growing weak and tingly. It became difficult to open jars and painful to hold either a cup of hot beverage or a glass of any iced drink. Clearly, the much-dreaded neuropathy was making its grand entrance in all of its glory. My body seemed to be getting more tired as everything that I tried to accomplish required more effort, more patience, and more inner strength. This cancer business is definitely not for the faint of heart! It is an ongoing battle with multiple components to defeat as the disease and the treatments take their toll on the body and fiercely try to sabotage the positive workings of the mind and the spirit. But with ten taxol treatments endured and only two more to go, Dave's optimism and encouragement were often heard in his motto to me of "Onward and upward—now let's go!" My Monday night Bible women offered the Scripture in Romans 5, verses 3 and 4 as my personal motto: "… But we also rejoice in our sufferings because we know that suffering produces perseverance; perseverance, character; and character, hope." And so we continued day after day in that glorious spirit.

27

Dave's E-Mail—June 21

Yay! Today we finished taxol! I refer to "we" because our friend and pastor, Asa Hunt, had counseled us early in this journey that this is *our* cancer, not just Sue's. We are a team in the effort and in the hope as we travel down this road together. Such sage advice that has helped me so much over these weeks and months. But it truly is *her* cancer—and what an amazing woman she is! How lucky can a guy be to have married such a woman, and after thirty-six years continue to be learning as I witness her strength and faith. God even looks out for and blesses sinners like me. Amazing grace!

Taxol treatments are finished and we are convinced that the tumor is gone. Thanks to the power of prayer and MD Anderson, we are breathing a little easier these days. An ultrasound on July 5, will confirm what we believe to be true. The battle "ain't" over, but we are giving it a heck of a run. Sue is such a trooper, but taxol has taken its toll. She hurts from muscle and nerve damage—sort of walks like an ancient Chinese woman with bound feet. Her toenails are about to fall off, but she sure is cute with her bald head and designer scarves!

Now we have two weeks before beginning the three-month protocol of a triple-whammy chemo called FAC. Taxol seems to have been such a success that we are actually looking forward to the new routine with this new drug. Sue had asked Dr. Cristofanilli if it was necessary to proceed with FAC since we will know shortly if the tumor is gone. He simply smiled at her and said, "See you on the fifth of July." Even if the tumor is gone, FAC will further battle any cells that might have escaped into her system. The side effects of nausea and hair loss might be more pronounced, although it will be difficult to determine the latter since she has no hair left to lose. I will miss our long days of the taxol treatment—that's when I got to whup her in gin rummy marathons while she was distracted by the bags of stuff dripping into her chest. FAC only takes a few hours once every three weeks.

Please don't forget her now—this is a long process and your prayers, cards, calls, and support are such a powerful force in the healing process. We feel and appreciate your love and prayers. Thanks to God for all of our blessings. Love, Dave.

28

From Laughter to Panic to Forgiveness

Laughter is so good for the body and the soul! It is refreshing. It is a stress-buster. It is a tonic to lift us out of the doldrums of life's more ominous circumstances. Some people laugh more easily than others. Dave's family can laugh with the best of them, but my family was always more serious and less spontaneous with frivolity and humor and lighthearted laughter.

Dave did his best to keep me laughing. He rented movies and tapes of Jack Benny, Amos and Andy, and George Burns. We went to the comedy theater. But his most unique effort was enrolling us in a comedy defensive driving course (we also received a ten percent discount on our insurance—the man is no fool). There we sat for seven hours in a small conference room of a mediocre motel with "offenders" (meaning traffic violators who had received tickets for their offenses), laughing at the jokes of a wannabe comedian who was actually quite funny as he extolled the virtues and mandates of careful and lawful road etiquette. Surely a strange way to spend a Saturday, but it truly did bring the desired effect. I was very grateful for Dave's continual support as day after day we muddled through the cancer journey together.

****
Laughter is so good for the body and the soul!
****

But the best laughter of all was being in the presence of darling little Jake. He was between twenty-one and thirty-four months during the year that I was in treatment. Such a great and spontaneous age! I was anxious that he would recoil from me after I had my head shaved, but in his innocence and with his sweet unconditional love, he simply laughed and said, "Ma Ma has no hair," and then quickly jumped into my lap and asked if I would read him a story. Every antic, every cute phrase that so spontaneously spewed from his little mouth, every giggle that erupted from his innocent inner being contagiously brought laughter to my lips and joy to my soul. Watching the silliness between him and his dad, which was accompanied by wide eyes and gaping mouths and uproarious laughter from both of them, filled me with a lightness of heart and so much pleasure. Sometimes I thought my heart would burst with happiness.

As the long days of a Houston summer marched slowly and oppressively across the calendar, my feet worsened and my hands became weaker. It became increasingly more difficult even to open the Ambien bottle with the childproof cap. I had gotten in the bad habit of simply leaving the bottle with the top ajar on the table next to the guest room's sleeper sofa, where I spent my nights.

It was the fourth of July, and I was so excited that Mike and Marla and Jake and Jim were coming to share the holiday with us to dine on scrumptious charcoal-grilled hot dogs, corn on the cob, and even a fancy red, white, and blue dessert which I had created for the occasion. I had bought a festive plastic tablecloth and colorful Independence Day balloons to go with the red plastic plates, blue cups, and white napkins. I even had candles for the dessert so that we could sing *Happy Birthday* to America and Jake could blow out the flames.

After they arrived, we spent a couple of hours with all of us enjoying Jake's world of laughter and fantasy, silliness and fun. Soon Marla took him upstairs to nap in his crib, which was in our guest room. Marla then donned a swimsuit and went outdoors to bask in the sunshine and cool off in the pool. Mike, Jim, Dave, and I settled comfortably in the family room relaxing, talking, and watching the Astros play ball. Isn't that what one is supposed to do on the Fourth of July? At one point, I thought I heard a noise from upstairs, but we all listened carefully and then determined it was nothing. A short time later, Jim asked me for a picture that he wanted to take home with him. The picture was upstairs, and I really didn't feel like climbing the stairs to search for it. My feet were hurting, I was tired, but I didn't want to disappoint Jim. So up I went.

Imagine my shock when I saw Jake standing in the doorway to our bedroom. He had never before gotten out of his cribs, neither this one nor the one at his own home. I said, "Jake, what are you doing?" He looked so serious, and then he took my hand. This precious twenty-six-month-old child, somehow knowing deep within himself that he had done something terribly wrong, led me into the room where I slept and pointed to the open bottle of sleeping pills. I said, "Jake, did you put any of those pills into your mouth?" He looked at me with such trust and with such a sad little face nodding his head yes. My heart stopped, but I remained calm as I poured the pills into my hand. It was a new prescription of thirty pills and I had consumed one the previous night, so I knew there should be twenty-nine pills in the bottle. There were twenty-five! (Even as I write this story more than four years after the fact, the panic and the fright rack my body and the tears flow down my face.)

****

Oh, my God, please don't let him die!

****

I yelled downstairs that I needed help. Mike and Jim flew up the stairs, taking them three at a time. I told them that it appeared Jake had swallowed four sleeping pills. Our peaceful day had just become a nightmare of confusion and fear. Jim called poison control and was told to get Jake to the hospital emergency room immediately. The three of them and Marla hurriedly left. Dave and I were alone, and I was hysterical! "How could I have been so totally negligent? It's my fault! Oh, my God, please don't let him die! How could I live if Jake dies? Mike and Marla must hate me!" These were my thoughts and hysterical outbursts as I paced the room sobbing and shouting and totally out of control.

The trauma of the cancer experience paled in comparison to the fear and anxiety and incredible panic that were now consuming my body and my soul. Dave grabbed me and slapped me to release me from my hysteria, and then held me as I quietly cried. It was then that I turned to God, kneeled in reverence, and prayed desperately that he would have mercy on this beautiful child. I was aware that I felt calmer, and as I became more rational, I began to sense a prodding urge to go back upstairs and determine where Jake might have wandered while he had been alone. So I went back upstairs to the room where Jake had found the pills. I noticed a few of his books which had been in his crib were now lying on the sofa. Perhaps he had been sitting there looking at his books when he discovered the open bottle. I picked up the books and there on the sofa was half of a pill. I knew then that at most he had ingested three-and-a-half pills. It then occurred to me that perhaps he had spilled the bottle, and so I frantically fell to my hands and knees to search the carpet, looking carefully under the sofa, but there were no pills.

As I was pulling myself up, I grabbed the cushions and thought that perhaps he had been playing with the pills and had been hiding them in between the pillows. I threw the cushions to the floor and there were the three other pills. I became hysterical again, but this time with elation and joy! I yelled to Dave to call the hospital and tell them that Jake had only ingested one half of a pill! We didn't know what was happening at the emergency room, but I was ecstatic and so grateful with the results of my search! With enormous relief in my heart, I went to my knees, laughing and crying and repeating, "Thank you, thank you, thank you!"

****

The peace that can only come from God follows my conversations with him.

****

In retrospect, I realize that it was only after I prayed that my physical being was calmed and I was able to think rationally. So many times this has proven true for me. The peace that can only come from God follows my conversations with him. And with that peace comes the ability to cope and to hope and to act. It is such a comfort to know that God listens to us and guides us if only we are open to receiving him so that we do not miss the signs he gives so freely to ease our burdens. I am deeply humbled by the gift and the blessing of knowing that God cares so deeply and walks with me in every occurrence in my life.

Jim called from the hospital and told us that our message hadn't reached them before the doctor had pumped Jake's stomach, but that he was doing just fine. After about three hours of observation, Jake was released and they all came home. I wasn't sure what Mike's and Marla's reaction toward me would be. But both of them hugged me and expressed that neither of them wanted me to chastise myself and dwell on what might have been. It was an accident and there was to be no blame. I was so relieved and grateful, but it took many weeks and a counseling session for me to finally let go of the guilt and the persistent thoughts of the potential horror of that day.

And so a day that had begun with so much anticipation and lots of silly fun ended in forgiveness and incredible understanding, humble appreciation of the fragility of life, and a heartfelt thanksgiving to God for his direction and mercy.

29

Why Me?

I've just been told by my doctor that the mammogram and ultrasound confirm that the tumor is gone! He says that the relatively short period of time required for the taxol to destroy the tumor leads him to conclude that there is probably no cancer left in my body. I am ecstatic with joy and gratitude. I hug him and we laugh the laughter of relief and excitement, and yet I feel anxious and sad. I can't shake the guilt and the reality of what could have been so tragic with Jake because of my negligence! And my mind won't let me forget the face of a young woman whom I knew as a teenager and heard today has been killed in an automobile accident.

****
Oh, God, why *me?* ... It is a mystery that I do not understand!
****

The incredible news about me is a moment for celebration, and yet when I get home, the tears flow like a river down my face. What about all of those men and women at MD Anderson and all over the world who long to hear the words that have just been delivered to me, but who never will? What about the family of a young woman in our church who was struck and killed by lightning two days ago? Oh, God, why *me?* Why *me?* Why have I been set free for this moment in time from the clutches of earthly death? Why will I live and others who have the same disease succumb to death? It is a mystery that I do not understand!

It consumes me for the next three days. I go to my Monday night Bible class, and as my friend Susan holds me in her arms, I sense the power and love of Jesus cradling me. I am struggling with the anxiety of waiting for endoscope results praying that I don't have esophageal cancer. The sebaceous cyst in my navel oozes and I can't begin the next round of chemo because of the infection; I must wait until after removal of the cyst. My legs burn and my toes ooze. I am now taking a drug for the neuropathy pain. A panic attack takes me to the emergency room of

MD Anderson in the middle of the night where I am surrounded by expression-less, wan faces—by sounds of pain, by looks of hopelessness and despair.

I'm going to live—the world is in pain.

I'm going to live—my body is a mess.

I'm going to live—I'm going to live!

Finally, after three days of confusion, guilt, and deeply fluctuating emotions, God releases me into the realm of reality, and I sense incredible freedom, excitement, joy, and gratitude for the precious gift of life which has been restored to me even amidst the circumstances which engulf and surround me. God has graced me these past few days by allowing me to accept my own pain and share with compassion in the pain of others as I simultaneously celebrate what is good.

I trust God, I trust God's plan for my life, and I trust that he has more for me to accomplish in ways that will reflect who he is—a God of love and compassion and mercy and grace.

At church yesterday, Asa Hunt said, "Take a step even though you hurt; take a step even though you are fearful; take a step even though you are tired. Take a step toward God and he will run to you."

My steps are slower these days, but my faith is strong! Hallelujah, I'm going to live!

30

Excerpts from E-Mails

July 18

Howdy y'all! For those of you in other parts of the country or the world, that's a big Texas greeting. I hope you are enjoying some vacation time this hot summer doing whatever it is you like to do.

The second phase of my chemo treatment has begun. I am now receiving a combination of three drugs, commonly called FAC. Two of the drugs are dripped into me at MD Anderson and the third one comes home with me in a fanny-pack with a pump which releases the drug into my venous catheter over a period of seventy-two hours. It is not exactly conducive to sleep, but since I have been told to take antinausea pills every four hours religiously around the clock for the first six days of each of the four cycles on this protocol, I don't expect to be having prolonged sweet dreams for several days each month. As one who is very much a rule-follower, I hear my obnoxious alarm clock resonate in my ears twice during each night in order to follow the prescribed regimen, which will hopefully prevent (or at least lessen) the agony of nausea and vomiting. It is definitely worth the inconvenience and lack of sleep because, for at least round one, I experienced no problem. Praise God!

I am now taking an antibiotic for the infection in my toes and fingers which has been disgusting and painful. I went to my friendly "butcher" foot doctor, and without any painkiller, he and his assistant literally carved my toenails and several fingernails off their beds. I am afraid that Dave will have permanent marks on his arm where I was digging into his flesh from that excruciating pain. And yet once the nails had been removed and my toes cleaned, my feet felt better than they had in a long time. But they sure look ugly. And I won't be dancing anytime soon.

I am daily reminded of and amazed at the blessings this illness has brought to me, and for me, and for others. I am often approached or e-mailed or phoned about people who have read my e-mails and found something in them that was helpful to their own personal trial. I am acutely aware of God's continual guidance, love, and sovereignty as I share his and my story with others. I am so blessed by the care and love I receive from Mike and Marla and Jim. And what would I do without Dave's optimism and tenderness and love? I am so strengthened by the thoughts and prayers and love that all of you send my way. The journey is long but I am healing in so many ways other than the cancer cure. The chains of the illness have actually led to more freedoms in my relationship with God, with Dave, with my children, and with others. So I am truly blessed. I will close with *shalom*—peace be with you—remembering that "nothing, not even life nor death, can separate us from the love of God" (Romans 8:38-39).

August 15

Hi to all,

The dog days of summer are upon us, but that means the beautiful days of autumn can't be far away. Do I sound like I am trying to hurry this year along? Perhaps I am.

As you are all aware, I find great strength, hope, and peace in God. And I know that God uses means other than just worship, Bible-reading, and prayer to offer those gifts to us, and to remind us of the power of faith. He often uses people. I would like to share the stories of two women, one whom I have never met. She is the sister of a friend, and her name is Sandy. The other woman is Lilly, whom we met in our first days at MD Anderson and who is going through the same treatment as I am. I have only been with Lilly for about ten minutes in person, but we talk on the phone to support one another. She lives in Louisiana and commutes to Houston for her chemo sessions. (I have mentioned her previously.)

****

… her life on earth has had meaning as a faithful child of God …

****

Sandy has been valiantly fighting ovarian cancer for five years. Ultimately it spread to her brain, and she has undergone surgeries, chemotherapy, and radiation in hopes of finding a cure. A few weeks ago, it was determined that the cancer has now spread to her liver, and six months of intense chemo followed by light chemo indefinitely is the course of treatment with no guarantees. Sandy is a woman of tremendous faith and has chosen not to go any further with treatment, but to live these next few months enjoying her family and preparing to go home to be eternally with God. She is at peace with her decision, and because of her faith, knows that she will be with her Lord and Savior forevermore. I so admire her courage and her faith. In a strange way, her story gives me encouragement and hope because she clearly understands that her life on earth has had meaning as a faithful child of God, and she rests in the knowledge of her eternal life.

Lilly has had some difficulty keeping her blood counts up during her taxol treatments. She had to miss a couple of sessions. I called her last evening only to find out that she was hospitalized for two weeks because her sugar count was over one thousand, and she was diagnosed with diabetes. She is also anemic from the chemo and is suffering from neuropathy in her feet. In the telling of her condition last night, all she could say was, "Praise God," and "I just thank God," and "God has been faithful," and "God heard her prayers and the prayers of others." I am blown away by the faith and the relationship both of these women have with God. It humbles me and gives me encouragement to continue to walk my own journey with God.

Two more treatments to go! One is on the twenty-eighth of this month and the last one in late September. I am doing so well—no nausea or mouth sores. I actually have white peach fuzz appearing on my head. Now that's exciting, to say nothing about the two hairs growing on my chin. Wow! I wouldn't admit that to just anybody, but you guys are all so special. The light grows brighter at the end of the tunnel. Praise God!

Let me close with a prayer that sustains me each day. It is called the Serenity Prayer:

"God, grant me the serenity to accept the things I cannot change, the courage to change the things I can, and the wisdom to know the difference."

Dave and I send our love and our prayers.

(Sandy died peacefully, surrounded and held by her family, just a few weeks after I wrote this e-mail.)

31

From Envy to Sorrow to Compassion

During Dave's work tenure with Shell in New Orleans from 1988 through 1997, we befriended a vivacious and beautiful woman named Cheryl. She was Dave's secretary for three years. Cheryl and her husband, who taught and coached men's basketball at a local school, had two wonderful children, Anthony and Melissa, whom we would see when we attended several basketball games over the years. Tall, thin, teenaged Anthony delighted to be in close proximity to his dad, the coach, and near the guys on the team, while shy, sweet Melissa preferred to sit in the bleachers close to her "Mommy," a term for her beloved mom that she never outgrew.

We moved back to Houston in 1997, and although we exchanged greetings through Christmas cards and a few phone calls, we ultimately began to lose touch.

Cheryl and I were diagnosed with breast cancer on the same day. Through word-of-mouth, we soon learned about our similar plight and were quick to reconnect and share the details of our personal journeys as we progressed through very different protocols. Cheryl initially had a lumpectomy, followed by four doses of chemo over a three-month period of time, and finished with a radiation protocol which took only one week to complete.

****

We laughed, we cried, we praised God for holding both of us in his tender care.
****

One August evening in 2001, Dave and I were anxiously awaiting Cheryl's knock on our door. She was in Houston on business and was coming to our home for dinner. She was completely finished with her treatments, and we could hardly wait to see her and embrace her with a congratulatory hug. She looked fabulous! Her skin was beautiful, her fingernails and toenails were polished in a gorgeous hue, her short black wig looked so natural and perky, her face was beaming with joy and excitement. We laughed, we cried, we praised God for holding both of us in his tender care. It was such a special reunion, and the three of us were warmed in our hearts and our souls by the intimate sharing of our lives through cancer. We understood the ravages of cancer, but we also relished in the truths of what cancer cannot do. It is so limited.

> It cannot cripple Love,
> It cannot shatter Hope,
> It cannot corrode Faith,
> It cannot destroy Peace,
> It cannot kill Friendship,
> It cannot suppress Memories,
> It cannot silence Courage,
> It cannot invade the Soul,
> It cannot steal Eternal Life,
> It cannot conquer the Spirit.
>   Anonymous

As Cheryl said good-bye that evening, my heart was so uplifted and I thanked God for her healing and for her presence in my life. Dave walked her to her car and I was left alone in the solitude for a few minutes. I literally sat down with a smile on my face and joy in my heart for the precious hours we had so enjoyed with this God-centered, gracious, gentle friend.

****
Was I truly jealous of Cheryl's toenails?
****

From out of nowhere, the tears slowly drifted down my cheeks. Oh, what a fine line separates our emotions! Suddenly I was sad and maybe even angry as my thoughts turned to me. As I looked at my ugly toenails and fingernails (or what was left of them), as I dwelled on the fact that Cheryl's treatment was already completed and I had yet to finish chemo, to say nothing about surgery and the six weeks of radiation therapy to follow, my body began to shake with uncontrollable sobs. What had just happened? How could I have been so joyful and genuinely excited for Cheryl just moments before and have now become such a sad, self-pitying, tired mass of tears?

Was I truly jealous of Cheryl's toenails? Was I coveting her successful and speedy recovery? The Bible tells us in Romans 12:15 to "mourn with those who mourn and rejoice with those who rejoice!" How easily I had allowed my own condition to overpower my elation for Cheryl! I quickly prayed that God would forgive my shallowness and self-absorption and grant me the peace and serenity to bask in Cheryl's great joy and rejoicing.

When Dave returned, he held me in his arms, sensing the reasons for my emotional state. He simply said, "It's okay, it's okay!" In his voice, I heard God say the same thing. I was calmed and soothed, and I knew that God had just answered my prayer request for peace and serenity. We went up to bed marveling at Cheryl's recovery, her attitude, her faith, and her beautiful nails.

Over the many months that followed, as I continued my battle, Cheryl and I spoke, but she did not reveal the pain that was currently tearing her apart. Her marriage had ended in divorce. Her world had been falling apart, but she did not want to burden me with her problems while I was still forging through my own. It was months after her divorce that she finally divulged her circumstances and shared her devastation at the breakup of her marriage. My heart broke for her, but I was awestruck at her dignity, her lack of bitterness, her forgiving heart. God had sustained her yet again through another emotional upheaval, and she praised the Lord.

Today, as I write this story, it is more than two years since Cheryl visited our home that evening when I allowed a petty jealousy to invade my heart. Today it is different. My heart is breaking with immense sadness, with consuming compassion, with deep sorrow. Four days ago, Cheryl buried her sweet, precious twenty-one-year-old daughter, Melissa. When I spoke with Cheryl today, she said, "Sue, my heart has been shattered forever!" Melissa had been shot in a random act of violence earlier this month, while Dave and I were vacationing in Canada, oblivious to the traumatic events that Cheryl and her family were enduring.

****

There is an ache in Cheryl's heart that is mammoth ....

****

Today Cheryl shared the contradictions of her heart during the days when she came to the realization that her beloved child was going to die. She was consumed by the devastation and the love, the horror and the peace, the frustration and the support, the helplessness and the tender moments, the desperate tears and the quiet reflections, the pain of loss and the comfort of faith. There is an ache in Cheryl's heart that is mammoth—a dark hole that causes her to weep and grieve and wonder why. But there is an incredible faith and trust in God which envelops her very soul. She is a testimony to God's love as she reveals how the peace of God has enfolded her as if she is safe and secure, wrapped in his loving arms. Her courage, her strength, her beautiful spirit—all gifts from God—are an inspiration to all who know her.

I have learned not to be envious of anything. But if I were to envy Cheryl, it would be for her obedient and faithful walk with God. Thank you for helping me to understand that although our physical bodies and our emotions can be ravaged and attacked and broken, our spiritual relationship with Jesus gives us the peace and the comfort and the courage to remain faithful to him on this journey called life. Thank you for allowing me to be a part of your life.

32

The Horror of Evil

I awaken to the joyful sounds of the chirping birds as they celebrate this day of sunshine and blue skies. I am happy! Today is Mike's birthday and I smile as I remember how gleeful and elated I was just moments after we greeted this miracle—a baby boy that Dave and I had named many years before when we were dating in high school and imagining a future together. I laughed and hugged the doctor's neck, introducing him to Michael David Teall. Without hesitation, in my giddiness (probably induced by the ether I had breathed during delivery), I asked the doctor when I could do this again. He just smiled at me like I was a little crazy and told me to get some sleep. That was so long ago, but the memory lingers precious and sweet in my heart.

I am happy as Dave hugs me good-bye and goes off for the day to attend two meetings; he acts as a facilitator as part of his volunteer work in the community. I watch him leave and am grateful that he has returned safely from a week's adventure tuna-fishing off the coast of California. I missed him while he was away, but was elated at a renewed sense of independence which had allowed me to trek to MD Anderson three times for my third FAC chemo treatment and the weekly changing of the dressing of my venous catheter port. I was relieved and excited that I truly had missed him for himself and not because he has been the prop upon which I have leaned so heavily these many months.

I am happy relishing the time I will share with my friend Susan today, as she is coming over for a light breakfast and meaningful conversation. As I greet her at the door, our neighbor and good friend, Bill, informs us that he has just heard on television that a passenger airline has crashed into the World Trade Center in New York. We all exclaim our disbelief and concern over that tragedy, but Susan and I decide to enjoy our time together for the next couple of hours knowing that we will hear more about this incredible accident later on the news. We don't turn on the television. I don't answer the phone as it rings three different times. The recorder will take the messages and I will attend to them later.

It is early afternoon. Susan has left. I pour myself a Diet Coke and turn on the television. Why are people frantically running through the streets of New York with a humongous cloud of smoke and ash and debris chasing them? What are these pictures of the Pentagon with gaping holes and fire, and why are the announcers talking about a plane going down in Pennsylvania? I am terrified when I see the plane crash into the World Trade Center—and then another. I panic! I feel weak in the knees and wonder if I might faint. I am confused and I am frightened to be alone.

****

The realization slowly sinks in that this country is no longer safe.

****

I call Bill and Carol and go next door to be with them. Soon I realize the significance and the horror, the helplessness and the compassion, the fear and the anger, the loss and the incredible sadness, the devastation and the agony, the incredible reality of this evil act. Tears become a way of life for many days. Depression rules our minds and the coverage occupies our waking hours. The realization slowly sinks in that this country is no longer safe. We are hated by those who want to cause us harm. Life as we have known it for more than two hundred years has changed. May God help us all!

Several days later, I write the following e-mail:

As we continue to walk through our daily lives, it remains inconceivable that such a horrific act of terrorism has staggered this country. Our hearts continue to ache for the victims and their families, the rescue workers and all who have lost a loved one or friend. Our faith in the goodness of humanity is strengthened when we hear about the kindnesses offered one to another in the city of New York as they struggle to repair their broken hearts and comfort their shattered souls.

Perhaps it is the perfect time for each of us to reflect on our own attitudes and behaviors when it comes to relationships with others. Perhaps we need to be asking God to forgive us for our anger, bitterness, jealousy, and envy toward our family members, friends, and neighbors. Perhaps we need to reflect on our own biases and judgments of others who are different from us. I pray that God would help me to overcome my insular heart.

****
… we often shun, reject, and even abhor the diversity
of race, color, culture, and religion.
****

I am reminded of a sermon Jim preached about diversity. He offered that as human beings we marvel and embrace the uniqueness, beauty, and individual properties of the vast variety of trees. We appreciate the colors, the sizes, the shapes, and special qualities of the elms, the aspens, the spruce, and the red buds. We are in awe when we witness the majesty and splendor of all of those trees living in community.

But when it comes to people, we often shun, reject, and even abhor the diversity of race, color, culture, and religion. How sad that as "aspens" or "spruce" we experience such conflict appreciating the similarities and the differences of those "trees" that do not replicate ourselves. How different the world would be if we could live harmoniously accepting and embracing the richness and beauty of diversity.

I am so encouraged by the rallying around our flag by all segments of our population and by the rallying around prayer by all faiths. Perhaps we can truly be united as a country in the face of this disaster, and begin to honestly care about and understand and forgive each other for wrongs and for misunderstandings and for not being respectful of all human beings—creations of God.

What can we do? Pray, pray, pray, pray for justice to be done. Pray for our leaders and for the leaders around the world to follow righteous ways of seeking justice for those who are responsible. Pray that light will conquer darkness, and good will overcome evil. And pray for all of those innocent lives that will surely be caught in the crossfire. It is time for warring parties all over the globe to learn the language of love rather than hate; to learn to give rather than take; to begin to respect rather than resent. In God we must trust! And to God we must pray!

33

Sixteen Roses

As I lie on this bed and concentrate on each drip progressing through the tube on its journey into my veins and through my body, I am overcome with emotion. This is the final chemo treatment of the protocol which I have been following for six months. I am elated because it appears the drugs have completed their incredible task—to rid my body of the cancer which threatened my very life. I smile to myself with relief. Dave and I hug and high-five. It is a milestone on the cancer path.

And there is such a deep appreciation within me for each man and woman who has treated me with incredible kindness and professionalism these many weeks as they administered the lifesaving drugs. They have created a comfort zone for me instead of a place to fear. We've laughed together and shared personal stories. Dave and I have so enjoyed discovering where each person was born and how long they have been affiliated with MD Anderson. I will always be grateful for their role in our adventure. As we leave the chemo area for the final time today, we hug them and thank them and know that we will truly miss their smiles, their support, and their gracious spirits.

There are three segments along this path for my treatment: chemo, surgery, and radiation. With chemo behind, I can now look forward with anticipation to the second phase. Dr. Cristofanilli, my oncologist, and Dr. Fred Ames, my surgeon, agree that I will undergo a lumpectomy with the additional removal of several nodes under my left arm. The date has been scheduled for October 31—is that some kind of a trick or will it turn out to be an amazing treat? For now, I have been given my freedom to relinquish all treatments for the next five weeks in order to rest and reenergize my body from the harshness of the chemo in preparation for the surgery.

We arrive home to find the most exquisite arrangement of sixteen gorgeous red roses. The card reads: "One rose for each chemo treatment you have so courageously endured." It was signed, "Love, Frank." They are from my ex-brother-in-law. How beautiful! How thoughtful! I stare at each glorious petal and I am touched. Sixteen rounds of chemo over six very long months. We did it! Praise God! This phase is *over!*

34

Modeling a Walk of Faith

Who is this young woman walking down the church aisle dressed in shorts and sneakers and a tee-shirt with—oh, my gosh, it's a picture of my face and bald head on the front of her shirt! I've never seen this person before! Who gave her that picture of me? I do not understand what is happening here!

My composed demeanor suddenly comes unglued as I sit in the front row. In a state of confusion, I watch this beautiful, smiling young woman approach the microphone.

It is a Sunday morning and I am about to speak to the congregation about the importance and relevance of the Women's Ministry programs as they have pertained to my life and faith journey. I feel honored and excited to share my insights as to the significance of God's ministry through these efforts of the Women's Ministry and how God's presence in Bible studies, retreats, special events, and service projects have impacted my life.

Our son Jim is the leader of this particular worship service, a contemporary service called Quest. He will be preaching in just a few minutes, and Dave and I will again be amazed at his wisdom, at his God-given ability to preach, at his grace and humility as he speaks about Jesus, our Lord.

Earlier this morning, before the service began, Jim had told me that he would introduce Bev, who would then introduce me. And now at the microphone, she tells the congregation that she is wearing this rather casual outfit because yesterday she participated in the Susan Komen Breast Cancer Race for the Cure in honor of me. I smile at her in gratitude, but don't allow my emotions to overcome me as momentarily I will need every bit of composure to give my testimony.

****

… she found the courage and faith and trust in God to confront her issues ….
****

Bev explains to the congregation how I have changed her life. What? How can that be? How could I have changed her life when I have never seen her before this moment? She continues by stating that Jim had shared all of my e-mails with her. She tells how conflicted, frightened, and uncertain she had been for many weeks as to how she should deal with a serious family problem and relationship. As she continued to read my e-mails, she found the courage and faith and trust in God to confront her issues and move forward in the healing process for her and her family. She thanked me for modeling a faith walk which gave her credence in the relevance of God in her situation.

She was grateful for the message that our courage, our strength, our trust, and our faith come directly from God when we open our hearts and our minds to receive him and to invite him into the circumstances of our lives. Scripture tells us that all things are possible with God (Matthew 19:26). Bev received that message in her heart and was able to face the confrontation in her life.

Bev invited me to come forward and we hugged, sharing an emotional, private moment publicly. As she returned to her seat, I thanked her and then I assured the congregation that I no longer looked like that picture on Bev's shirt. Under the wig that adorned my head, I was sporting a quarter inch "do" of pure white fuzz. The laughter broke the poignancy and the power of the precious moment that Bev and I shared. I took a deep breath and then I spoke.

Jim preached. We all prayed and sang and worshipped God. What a glorious morning, and yet another gift from God!

For many days I contemplated what the experience with Bev meant for me. As I reflected over these many months, I was keenly aware that she was not the first person to relate to me how my story with God and with cancer had impacted his or her life or the life of someone to whom my e-mails had been forwarded. Each time I was amazed and humbled that perhaps God was using me in some profound way. What an incredibly awesome thought! Was my niece, Linda, correct when she so astutely said that my purpose as I journeyed through cancer was to relate God's story of his love, his grace, and his mercy as evidenced in my life? The idea is humbling, even terrifying. Where will this lead? What are God's plans for me?

****

What I *couldn't* seem to shake was the "still small voice"….

****

Over the next eighteen months I was often asked if I would consider writing a book about my experience with God through cancer. I would smile and thank the person for his or her interest, but quickly let the idea slip from my conscious thought.

What I *couldn't* seem to shake was the "still small voice" deep within my soul that was subconsciously urging me and perhaps commanding me to indeed relate the physical, emotional, and spiritual journey which had dominated my life for a full year. Was this the voice of God? The thought of revisiting the painful and frightening experiences on the journey seemed more than I wanted to bear. As the months steadily slipped away, I became certain that God was the author of the message that would not leave me alone. I began to believe that it was indeed his will that I should write this story.

In April 2003, I attended a two-day workshop at Rice University. I learned the process for creating a nonfiction book. I delayed another three months rejecting what I knew in my heart was God's will for me, but fearful of the return visit to 2001, and uncertain as to my own ability and stamina to undertake such a project.

In July 2003, I succumbed to "the call" and opened the journal in which I had written about my experiences and feelings during that incredible year. (I find it interesting that I had never written a journal before that time nor have I since.) I slowly read five or six entries and allowed myself to "let go" and reexperience each moment of those passages written from my own hand and heart so long ago. I wept uncontrollably and cried out to God, "Why do you want me to suffer through that difficult time all over again?" I put the journal away, told Dave that I just could not do it, bowed my head to "explain" to God, and in that very moment knew that I would in fact obey his will.

It became so clear to me that my intense reaction to the reading of my own words was the special gift from God that would allow the writing to flow from my heart and my soul and not just from my memory. I needed to feel the experience in order for it to be genuine. I laughed through fresh tears comprehending without a doubt that just as God had accompanied me on the original journey, he would be the director that would humbly allow me to reflect on his and my story.

When Dave asked me how I was going to initiate the story, I laughed confidently and said sincerely, "I don't have a clue, but I trust God will pave the way!" I went into my room, sat down with a legal pad of paper, invited God into my space, prayed that he would give me the words to say, and I began to write!

35

If the Shoe Fits, Wear It

With fear and anticipation, I walk into Brucettes, a specialty shoe store in Houston. The fear is that I won't find shoes to fit my nerve-damaged feet and the hopeful anticipation is that I will. The days are getting cooler and I am desperate to be rid of the shoes I have worn for over six months—a pair of black sandals which are the only shoes in my closet my feet can tolerate. A few weeks ago I did purchase a pair of sneakers two sizes larger than my feet in order to give my toes ample room to seek comfort. Dave laughingly says that if the flood ever comes, we'll be okay. He'll hop into one sneaker, I'll hop into the other, and we'll just drift along like Old Mother Hubbard. They really are obnoxious and don't exactly look very chic with my church duds.

So today I am greeted by Bill, the shoe salesperson, who immediately seems to comprehend my situation and enthusiastically disappears in search of the perfect glass slippers. While he is on a mission in the stockroom, I wander around the store and "oooh and aaah" over the beautiful, stylish shoes which will not today be introduced to my feet nor find a home in my closet. I will be so content to find a pair that will replace my overused black sandals and my humongous sneakers.

Bill returns several times with boxes of potential purchases. He carefully tends my feet and we try a multitude of shoes. He patiently and graciously involves himself in this emotional moment for over ninety minutes, and when he closes the final box, I have selected nine pairs of shoes. I am deliriously happy and so relieved and so grateful. Bill senses the importance of what this means for me, and with tears in both of our eyes, we hug.

I know that Dave will think that I have gone slightly overboard (perhaps I have), but it has been so very long since I have felt the desire to purchase anything for myself. I haven't had the energy or the inclination to shop. Today, I did.

I feel like Imelda Marcos of the Philippines, who was reported to have over a thousand pairs of shoes. Such extravagance! My eleven pairs (the nine new ones, the beat up sandals, and the "boats") don't even come close, yet today I feel like

Cinderella. I can hardly wait to step out in one of my new wildly extravagant purchases. You know what they say: "If the shoe fits, wear it!"

36

Pretend That You Are Fasting for Jesus

I woke this morning to glorious sunshine, tender greetings of encouragement and love from Dave, and a smile on my face reflecting on the news that my niece Tammy and her husband, Dave, shared with us the previous evening. Tammy said that she wanted me to face surgery with a positive and exciting sense of life. She told us that she and Dave were pregnant and the happy blessing was due in May. Wow—another precious life to love! I felt joyful, refreshed, renewed, excited, and full of hope for the future. Birth, life, death—a beautiful and miraculous continuity established by God. For God delivers us at birth, he sustains us through life, and we return to him at our earthly death. I am overjoyed with thanksgiving and praise when I reflect on the awesomeness of that cycle.

As we entered MD Anderson, my mood was joyful and upbeat. I felt no fear, confident on this Halloween that this day would truly be the beginning of the end of my cancer journey. Due to a scheduling error, my surgery was delayed, so Dave and I found ourselves with time on our hands. We went to the patient welcome center and came face-to-face with a couple who were new to the system; she had just been diagnosed with breast cancer. During a conversation, we watched their demeanors change from fear and uncertainty to a sense of peace and confidence as Dave and I shared our story with them. They couldn't believe how calm and jovial we were as I was about to surrender to the knife—the second stage of the protocol. They thanked us for being a blessing to them of hope and courage and triumph.

Around noon, I was prepped for surgery in a very specific manner. In order for the surgeon, Dr. Fred Ames, to know exactly where he was to proceed, the location of the tumor had to be precisely marked on my skin. This involved a new mammogram which would then mirror image previous mammograms so that pins could be inserted into my breast at the precise location. It seemed simple enough, but because of a couple of miscues, I was attached to the vise grips of the mammogram machine for thirty-five minutes while a kindly nurse gently reminded me every few seconds not to move and to breathe normally. Easy for her to say! I felt enormous relief when my breast was finally released from the clutches of that machine. What followed brought comic relief as a Styrofoam coffee cup was taped over the pins so that they would not inadvertently be knocked out of their "home" stuck in my breast. Dave and I couldn't help but laugh at the reality of this very professional and sophisticated medical facility embracing a Styrofoam cup as part of its medical paraphernalia.

How could this beautiful Jamaican aide, who was pushing my wheelchair toward the surgical location, know that I would be comforted by her words? Marilyn simply stopped transporting me, bent down in front of me, took both of my hands, smiled her most gorgeous and effervescent smile, and quietly whispered that she knew that I would be okay because she knew that God was with me. We hugged for a brief moment. I thanked her for her encouragement and her precious words. I told her that I would return tomorrow to give her a big hug so that together we could celebrate victory.

****

"Pretend that you are fasting for Jesus—it will take the hunger pains away."
****

The nurse assigned to me in pre-op was such a delight. She excitedly informed me that I was her very final patient in a twenty-five year career. Her enthusiasm and joy about retirement was effervescent and we jokingly told her to make sure her mind was on me during the next few hours and not on her dreams of retirement. She laughed and assured me that I was her only focus. I mentioned (probably whined) about how hungry I was since it was approaching nineteen hours since any sustenance had crossed my lips in pursuit of my stomach. This is not good for the gal who likes her three square meals every day. She smiled, held my hand, and softly said, "Pretend that you are fasting for Jesus—it will take the hunger pains away." Our eyes held for a brief moment. I sank into a deep relaxation and said, "Thank you. You just made my day." And I knew that this lovely nurse, who obviously loved God, would have her mind solely and properly focused on my behalf while I was her patient. Another gracious gift from my Lord!

The surgeon joked about being late. It was his day to pick up his young twins from school and he had been delayed. I couldn't help but take comfort in this renowned physician at MD Anderson sharing his delight in his children. Somehow his genuineness made me feel more connected to him as a parent and a human being.

By the time the anesthesiologist was ready to sedate me, I felt tranquil and special and tenderly cared for. I was ready to let go and surrender to these professionals so they could perform their skills on my behalf. I was confident that the Styrofoam cup would surely be an obvious clue for Dr. Ames as to where he should place his knife. I closed my eyes in peace and as I was losing consciousness, I wondered if Tammy and Dave would be blessed with a boy or a girl.

The lumpectomy surgery lasted more than three hours, but I returned to my full senses (well, that's probably debatable) rather quickly in recovery. Dave and I were told that the procedure had gone very well. There was no sign of any tumor in the breast, and that surrounding tissue had been sent to pathology. Dr. Ames had also performed a procedure under my left arm pit removing much of the "fat pack" where the nodes reside. That too would be studied by pathologists. We would have the results in a few days.

For some unknown reason, I was moved to the VIP section of the hospital where I occupied a room that was the equivalent of a very fine hotel room. I felt like a queen as I settled in for the overnight stay. I was given a light supper which I consumed rather quickly and enjoyed as if I were at a gourmet restaurant. Jim popped in to give me a hug and a thumbs up. I spoke to Mike and Marla and Jake on the phone. Dave simply smiled and held my hand. Our hearts were so full of gratitude and praise.

The night nurse said that she would not disturb me for vitals during the night, but would perform that duty should I call her for any reason. The morphine machine was next to my bed so that I could control my own pain medication. How cool is that! I slept amazingly well even though I was attached to a drain protruding from my left side allowing the waste fluids to flow into a container which would be measured twice daily for several days to determine when my body was ready to assimilate the remainder of the fluids on its own. The pain was bothersome, but not excruciating. The venous port had been left in my right chest (since March) in the event that I would need further surgery as indicated by the results of the pathology report. I felt rather bulky and cumbersome, but at the same time, I sensed myself unshackled and free. The cancer was no longer making me a prisoner in mind and body. The journey wasn't over, but I was no longer feeling the overwhelming burden which had been so prevalent for so long. In the silence of the night, each time I woke, I thanked God for all of his goodness—all of the love—all of the care that was being showered upon me from so many sources.

****
Our hearts were so full of gratitude and praise.
****

When morning dawned, I rose to the sound of the breakfast delivery. After relishing each morsel, I dressed and informed the nurse that I was going for a walk. There was a certain person whom I needed to see. I slowly meandered my way through the maze of hallways (which seemed like twenty miles), where amidst the thousands of patients and staff dealing with fear and pain and death there is such an overwhelming aura of joy and faith and life. When I reached my destination, there she was—almost as if she knew I'd be there at that precise moment. I beamed at my new friend, Marilyn, and said, "I told you that I would return today so that we could share this victory together." She smiled, we hugged, and amidst our mutual tears, she repeated over and over, "Praise God! Praise God!"

Today is the first day of the rest of my life. I feel great!

37

I Am Cancer-Free

What a beautiful November day! The sun is shining, the air is cool and crisp, the sky is blue and my heart sings of praise and thanksgiving and joy. Dave has gone for a morning walk in the park and I am alone in my solitude, watching the flames in the fireplace dance across the wood, mesmerizing me with their movement and light. My heart is at peace, yet I am excited because my entire family will arrive in several hours to celebrate this wonderful Thanksgiving holiday. So many of them offered to host this family meal today, but I insisted that I was up to the challenge and eager to have all of them with us in our home for this very special day of thanksgiving.

Soon I will prepare the dressing and stuff the turkey, bake two pumpkin pies, set the table for thirteen, make the orange-cranberry sauce, and peel the potatoes. But for the moment I simply relish my joy and my solitude with God. I open my hymnal in the quiet of the moment and I heartily sing, "For the Beauty of the Earth," "Now Thank We All Our God," "This is the Day that the Lord Has Made." I sense God's presence and I humbly pray.

I close my eyes and reflect on the happenings of the past three weeks while recuperating from the surgery. I smile to myself when I recall Dave patiently and methodically, with much humor and sarcasm, twice daily removing and measuring the fluid which drained from my side for several days (which seemed like weeks). We were both so ecstatic when the amount of fluid was finally considered low enough that the drain could be removed from my body with the expectation that my system could absorb whatever fluid continued to flow. (This turned out not to be the case. I had to return to MD Anderson for several weeks to have the area aspirated to drain the built up fluid which was causing pain. After three months, my body finally decided to cooperate and my aspiration days came to an end. Thank God!)

****

I laugh as I recall little Jake aping my every move ....
because he wants to share in my road to recovery.

****

I return upstairs to my room to complete the exercises which I faithfully exe-
cute twice daily in order to regain range of motion in my left arm and stretch the
muscles and tendons which had been cut during surgery so they don't atrophy. I
laugh as I recall little Jake aping my every move with his own little arm because
he wants to share in my road to recovery. How precious he is and how blessed we
are to have this mutual devotion to each other.

When I sit to rest, I am aware that the e-mail I sent just a few days ago to family and friends is in my reach. I begin to read my own words and I sense the emotion of the past nine months expressed in this message:

November 14

Nine months ago, I anxiously awaited a phone call that ultimately would tell me
that I had breast cancer. I will never forget the peace that enveloped me at that
exact moment knowing that it was the peace of God. I knew that I was turning
my illness and my life over to God, and I felt his assurance that he would take me
on this journey and bring me out whole on the other end (although I didn't
know what "whole" would look like). During these nine months, I have had my
ups and downs. I have laughed and I have cried. I have carried on the best that I
knew how—by trusting God. But I had a few pity parties along the way. I have
been nervous about infected toes and a sebaceous cyst. I have felt anxiety over
neuropathy in my feet and pains in my chest from the acid reflux made worse by
the chemo. I have worried about a colonoscopy, an endoscope, blurry vision, a
mind that seemed to "slip" for a short time and other annoying problems—all of
which have improved immensely over the past few weeks. But I have always
maintained a sense of peace about the cancer, and I thank God for that! For it
was only the grace of God that allowed nervous me to rest in the assuredness that
I felt he had imparted to me on that first day.

This morning I waited again for the phone call that would tell me the results
of the pathology report. I was a tad anxious, but nothing like I was those many
months ago. When my doctor called, he said that I am cancer-free. Hallelujah!
There isn't any evidence of tumor in the breast nor is there any cancer in the surrounding tissue. The "fat pack" which was removed by the surgeon was found to
have contained twenty-seven nodes and two of those had cancer cells remaining,

but the walls of those two appear unbroken allowing the doctors to assume that no cancer has escaped into my system. Dave and I pressed Dr. Cristofanilli by asking him if this meant there was no cancer left in my body. He affirmed by repeating that I am cancer-free!

****

Joy for me and sadness for others intertwine ....

****

Needless to say, it is a happy moment. It is filled with prayers of thanksgiving and glory to God. It is filled with tears of joy and also of pent up emotion for the long journey. It is filled with the humbleness of knowing how many people were praying for me and caring for me and encouraging me along the way.

I do not begin to know why I have been given a clean bill of health when so many never hear those words. It is a part of my tears. Joy for me and sadness for others intertwine and bring forth such a mixture of emotion. All I truly know is that I look forward to the continuation of my life, and prayerfully seek ways in which I can reach out to make a difference in a hurting world.

We meet with Dr. Cristofanilli next week to discuss the third step of the treatment—radiation. The journey continues, but with victory in sight. Today I had the central venous catheter removed. I had grown attached (figuratively and literally) to this piece of equipment which had been the pathway for the chemo to enter my body and do its job. I thanked it for a job well done, but almost jumped for joy when it was removed and I was told that I could shower in two days. I have not had a shower since March 30! *I can't wait!* Neither can Dave—ha ha!

We wish you a happy Thanksgiving; you are in our thoughts and prayers, and we love y'all.

I finish reading the e-mail and I am aware that tears are cascading down my cheeks. But I laugh out loud when I recall that first shower just a few days ago. Oh, how I relished that moment when I stepped into falling drops of warm water, allowing each droplet to gently caress and cleanse my entire body. I wanted to stay in the warmth of that cocoon forever. Such a simple event that we all take so much for granted, but, oh, what a precious gift!

My reverie is interrupted by the familiar sound of Dave's voice as he calls upstairs, "When are you going to start cooking the turkey and baking the pies?" I smile to myself realizing that some things never change, and I thank God for that and for Dave. "I'm coming." And I can hardly wait!

38

The Grand Entrance

I don't know what to do! Should I wear my wig or should I finally allow myself to be seen publicly with the fuzzy white down that is sprouting all over my head? I pace almost frantically in front of the mirror trying to determine if I have the guts and the self-confidence to face the multitudes of friends and acquaintances in my au natural look at the church Christmas luncheon which I am about to attend. "Come on, Sue. Make a decision," I say out loud.

Why am I so upset? I am suddenly startled at my own anxiety over this egoistic moment. I feel ashamed that I have allowed myself to think so shallowly about others and so vainly about myself. Am I actually entertaining the arrogant thought that people will reject or accept me because of my hairdo or lack thereof? How dare I be so presumptuous about the reactions of my church community which has consistently shown me grace, mercy, compassion, empathy, and support these many months? I walk out my door at peace with my decision and happily sense the cold air on my (almost) bald head.

Because I have procrastinated in front of the mirror most of the morning, I arrive slightly late and everyone is already seated. As I enter, I realize that my table is at the opposite side of the room. So now I have no choice but to make a grand entrance, assuring that everyone will be aware that I am not only late, but that my wig is not accompanying me. As I cross the room, people are smiling at me and some are actually silently clapping as I pass by their tables. I am greeted with hugs and tears as people leave their places to come over and greet me. One of the pastors holds me and quietly whispers, "I know that this took guts, but you look beautiful!" Whew! Another lesson learned along this journey in humility. How grateful I am! Thank you, God. And bye-bye, wig and hats and scarves. I don't need you anymore. Thanks for your services, but now I am free to be me!

39

Let the Burn Begin!

It is mid-December and I have rested and recuperated from the surgery. I am going to physical therapy twice weekly to stretch the muscles and the tendons under my arm where the twenty-seven nodes were removed. Tightness and pain are prevalent, but the therapy helps. I live in dreaded fear of edema (swelling) in my left arm which would be difficult to reduce because of the lack of lymph nodes. So I happily march myself down to MD Anderson and grunt, moan, and groan while the physical therapist pulls, tugs, and rubs my soreness.

The third round of treatment, radiation (otherwise known as "The Burn"), is the next stop on my journey and is about to begin. Dave and I have met with Dr. Elizabeth Bloom, the radiology oncologist, whom I found to be gentle but firm and very professional. She precipitated a moment of humor when I questioned whether to radiate the nodes in my neck region. I had heard that radiation in that area could foster the much-dreaded swelling in my arm. She smiled and said, "There are two reasons to radiate that area. The first is your possible demise!" Dave and I were momentarily taken aback, and then Dave jokingly said, "Well then, I guess there really is no need to hear reason number two." We all laughed heartily and the rapport among us was established. Dr. Bloom explained the procedure that will occur for the next six weeks, five days a week, for a total of thirty radiation treatments.

My chest was dissected into a geometric pattern of blue and red inks, with *X*'s and other meaningful marks to instruct the technicians who will oversee the actual radiation procedure. My chest looks like the chart of a basketball coach drawing up the play for the team's critical last-minute attempt to win the game.

So let the "burn" begin! I am eager to start the final phase of the treatment for this insidious disease called cancer which has so preoccupied my body, my mind, my spirit, my conversation, and my time for so long. But oh, how I pray that somehow my redheaded, fair skin will *not* burn badly enough to cause any problems. For, I can truly begin to smell and taste the finish line of this incredible race to defeat the enemy.

40

The Christmas Message

Christmas was quickly approaching and I had done little in preparation for its arrival. My brother, Jeff, and his wife, Rachael, were hosting the festive family dinner this year, so I was relieved of that particular preparation. My energy level seemed to be waning because of the daily radiation treatments. I was struggling to generate the excitement to go shopping for the family gifts, an activity I eagerly look forward to each year. I am not an enthusiastic shopper eleven months of the year, but have always loved the joy of purchasing and giving gifts at Christmas.

To my rescue came my dear friend, Mary Ellen—bless her heart—who said she needed to attack the mall and asked if I would go with her. With rather a long list in my pocket, I happily jaunted off with Mary Ellen to our destination, where every person in Houston was shopping that day. She proceeded to map out a strategy which would require the least amount of walking for me, handle some of my sales transactions while I rested, carry most of my packages, and, oh yeah, purchase the one item that was on her list. It became obvious that it was not necessary for Mary Ellen to go to the mall for herself that day; she went specifically to help me get my Christmas in order.

The Christmas season is a time of mixed emotions for many of us. The message of Christmas is one of peace, love, joy, and hope. It is one of reconciliation to God and to one another. But it doesn't always play out that way in individual and communal lives. I have personal memories of wonderful Christmas times centered on the birth of Christ, with family and friends and great food and special traditions. But I also have memories that evoke sadness and pain when Christmas was affected by family feuds and joyless meals and unspoken anger. Mary Ellen's act of kindness remains a joyful reminder in my heart of the true message of Christmas.

****

The story that little Jake knew so well about the first Christmas was coming to
life before his very eyes, and his soul was responding with glee.

****

On Christmas Eve day, Dave and I were blessed as both of our sons, our
daughter-in-law, and our precious grandson attended the service at First Presbyterian Church deemed appropriate for small children. I could not take my eyes
away from Jake as he responded with his entire being to the story of Jesus' birth.
There were live animals, children dressed as angels, the crèche with Joseph and
Mary, and a precious infant portraying the baby Jesus. There was a shining star
and the sound of trumpets and the shepherds abiding in the fields. The story that
little Jake knew so well about the first Christmas was coming to life before his
very eyes, and his soul was responding with glee. Such joy, such wonder, such
excitement, such purity and love appeared in that sweet little face as Jake lived the
special moment of the birth of his Lord, Jesus! I was swept away by the awareness
of the power of the love of God reflected in the face of this precious child. I
prayed that all peoples around the world might be able to sense that same love of
God in the faces, be they dark-skinned or light, of children around the globe.
Now, wouldn't that be the best gift of all?

41

It's Over—Praise God!

Oh, how I relished the thought of the New Year! We toasted with friends and family, we wore funny hats and blew crazy noisemakers. We watched the ball drop in Times Square and kissed the year farewell. 2001 was history, and from every indication, so was my cancer.

I still had four more weeks of radiation treatments and several more workouts with physical therapy, which were both taking their toll. I was tired most of the time. I contracted the flu and felt miserable, but I never missed a day of radiation over the six-week period. I knew in my heart and in my mind that the journey was nearly complete and that victory was in sight. But my physically abused body was totally spent. I accomplished very little during that final month. It took every ounce of my strength to haul myself daily out of the recliner and into the car, drive the twenty-five minutes to the radiation clinic, wait my turn, get zapped, and then drive the twenty-five minutes back home.

The staff at the MD Anderson radiation facility was wonderful (even though they inadvertently gave me the flu). One of the radiation therapists had a delicious sense of humor and kept me laughing. But I was particularly enamored with a young man who would read his Bible when he wasn't working with a patient. He was so gentle and compassionate. His name was Brad Tillman.

The last Friday in January 2002, marked my final treatment. My sensitive skin had survived the onslaught of radiation relatively intact. I lay down on the sterile machine to which my body had become so conformed and awaited the final zap. I was absolutely still as I listened to my own thoughts. My heart was so full of relief and release from all of the emotions of the past year. I was alone with my God and so humbly grateful.

****

And then it was over!

****

102

When Brad stepped into the room, he smiled, took my hand and said, "Just one more!" And then it was over! I felt the warmth of my tears cascading down my cheeks. I looked at Brad; his eyes were moist. I simply said, "Praise God!" As he assisted me to a sitting position, I thanked him for helping me through these weeks and wished all of God's good blessings for him and his wife, who was pregnant with their first child.

Before he left the room, I asked him what he was reading in the Bible and he said, "Funny that you should ask, because the verse reminds me of you. I was reading about the apostle Paul telling Timothy, 'I have fought the good fight, I have finished the race, I have kept the faith'" (2 Timothy 4:7). Brad could not have given me anything more special than those words of Holy Scripture as the finale to my long and arduous journey through breast cancer. We hugged and said good-bye. I exited my way out of the clinic and out of the vise grip of the cancer that had so impacted my life for one whole year.

Dave was waiting for me when I returned home. I was exhausted, but elated. We high-fived and kissed, laughed and cried. It was truly over. And we had won!

The doorbell rang. Standing outside were our dear friends Bill and Carol, with grins on their faces like Cheshire cats. Bill was holding a bottle of champagne, but our giddiness and joy had nothing to do with the anticipated bubbles. It was such a lovely celebration.

Amidst our zealous jubilation they confessed that together they had prayed for me every single night, from the alpha to the omega of my cancer experience. Dave and I were speechless, overwhelmed, and so very grateful for all of their care, their concern, and most especially for their prayers.

We toasted again—to the mysterious ways of God, to lasting friendship and to good health in the years to come.

****

… almost as if he were singing, "Ma Ma is cancer-free!"

****

Soon other friends and family arrived for a pizza celebration. Such a joyful, festive time we all shared! Dave had created a large sign on the computer which read "CANCER-FREE" and hung it, in glorious splendor, over the fireplace. Jake loved the sign and kept repeating, almost as if he were singing, "Ma Ma is cancer-free! Ma Ma is cancer-free!" Oh, what music to my ears—the reality of that truth coming from that sweet, precious child with whom I can hopefully share many, many more years to come. Praise God!

Epilogue

Wow! It has been over six years since that memorable morning in the shower when I discovered that "nasty little tumor" which dramatically altered our lives for a year.

But life has a way of moving forward despite the unexpected detours and bumps in the road. I thank God for new journeys, quiet reflections, and future anticipations. I am grateful for each new sunrise and I delight in the possibilities of each new day.

Dave and I have been blessed with two additional precious grandsons. Jake will be eight this year, Josh is three, and Justin was born in October 2006. We relish the moments we share with them. Watching them run and play and laugh and coo and smile and pray allows us to experience their childhood innocence of pure happiness.

I am eager to report that my friend and cancer buddy, Ronnie, continues to be cancer-free in Florida. I regret that I haven't seen her in a long time, but her voice on the other end of the phone brings me such joy and laughter. Way to go, Ronnie!

Cheryl experienced the trauma of yet another tragedy when Katrina forced her out of her water-logged home. Shell relocated her to Houston. In God's inexplicable timing, we all celebrated and praised God when she was able to purchase the home we were selling in order to move closer to our three little J's. It brings all of us such comfort and peace knowing that Cheryl occupies a space which we had previously so enjoyed.

Lilly and Vernon continue to reside in Louisiana and make the trek to Houston for her checkups at MD Anderson every six months. Lilly is excited about her daughter's upcoming marriage and continues to glorify God for all the blessings in her life. Her spirit and praise of the Lord are music to my ears.

Dr. Cristofanilli has had much success in his research on inflammatory breast cancer. His accomplishments have allowed MD Anderson to recently open a clinic for women suffering with this particular kind of cancer. I am so proud of his work and his dedication to finding the answers that will one day eradicate this insidious disease of breast cancer.

****

"My grace is sufficient unto you."

****

I continue to experience neuropathy in my feet and legs, but it doesn't stop me from walking three miles in forty-eight minutes. It is simply a constant reminder that I am alive. I think of the thorn in the side of the apostle, Paul (2 Corinthians 12:8-9). Jesus did not remove the thorn which plagued Paul, but rather said to him, "My grace is sufficient unto you." In other words, "I am what you need!"

Those words ring truer to me because of the cancer experience. And because I so believe that God's grace, mercy, love, and forgiveness through my Lord, Jesus, are truly what I need most in my life, I choose to share that with others through Bible studies and through this story of God's faithfulness. "May the grace of the Lord be with all of you as it is with me."

978-0-595-43675-0
0-595-43675-7